√ T5-AFO-235

GASTRO-INTESTINAL PROBLEMS

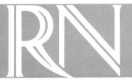

NURSING ASSESSMENT SERIES
JULIE MULL STRANGE, R.N., CCRN

Series Editor
Margaret Van Meter, R.N.
Clinical Editor, RN Magazine

MEDICAL ECONOMICS BOOKS
Oradell, New Jersey 07649

Library of Congress Cataloging in Publication Data

Strange, Julie Mull.
    Gastrointestinal problems.

    (RN nursing assessment series ; 4)
    Bibliography: p.
    Includes index.
    1. Gastrointestinal system — Diseases — Nursing.
I. Title.   II. Series: RN nursing assessment series ;
v. 4. [DNLM: 1. Gastrointestinal Diseases — nursing.
WY   100   R627   1982   v.4]
RC817.S77   1984   610.73'69   84-9106
ISBN 0-87489-285-6

Cover design by Jerry Wilke

ISBN 0-87489-285-6

Medical Economics Company Inc.
Oradell, New Jersey 07649

Printed in the United States of America

To my husband, Bill, for all his encouragement and patience

ACKNOWLEDGMENTS

Two people at the Maryland Institute for Emergency Medical Services Systems deserve special thanks. Elaine P. Rice of the Editorial/Publications Office provided much support and assistance in preparing the manuscript for publication. Paula M. Kelly, R.N., contributed the photographs for Figures 3-1, 3-8, 3-9, and 3-12.

CONTENTS

PUBLISHER'S NOTES

Physical assessment is an integral part of the nursing process. Sharpening assessment skills, therefore, is bound to add logic and reason to planning, intervention, and evaluation. This volume in the *RN Nursing Assessment Series* focuses on assessment of gastrointestinal function. It provides norms against which to compare pathologic findings.

For easy access, an outline format combined with a clear, concise text — an organizational scheme that has proven popular with nurses — was adopted. The illustrations, both halftone and line art, were selected specifically to add to the book's clarity and utility. Finally, the presentation of learning objectives and the inclusion of chapter quizzes, additional test questions, and a glossary make this book a learning/teaching tool.

Julie Mull Strange, R.N., CCRN, is Clinician II in the admitting area of the Shock Trauma Center at the Maryland Institute for Emergency Medical Services Systems in Baltimore. She is the author of a chapter on abdominal trauma in *Trauma Nursing* (Medical Economics Books, 1984) and of articles on nursing assessment of abdominal problems in *RN* Magazine. She has presented several classes and workshops on these subjects. Margaret Van Meter, R.N., the series editor, is *RN* Magazine's clinical editor for development and also serves as a private nurse consultant.

1

Anatomy and Physiology

OBJECTIVES

After completing this chapter, you will be able to:

1. List the basic functions of each organ of the gastrointestinal (GI) system

2. Describe the "arteries supplying and veins draining each organ"

3. List the secretion(s) of each organ.

A. Esophagus

1. Location

The esophagus, which lies behind the trachea, extends from the end of the laryngopharynx, through the esophageal hiatus in the diaphragm, and ends in the upper portion of the stomach (Figure 1-1).

Figure 1-1 *Anterior view of the structures in the GI tract*

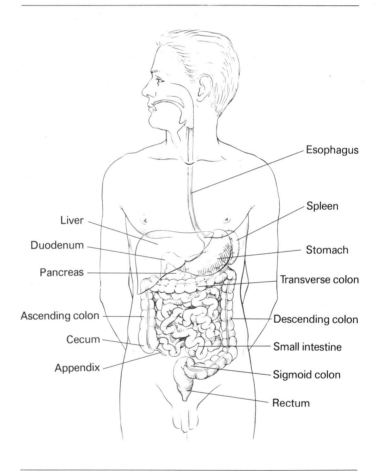

- Esophagus
- Spleen
- Liver
- Duodenum
- Pancreas
- Stomach
- Transverse colon
- Ascending colon
- Cecum
- Appendix
- Descending colon
- Small intestine
- Sigmoid colon
- Rectum

2. Description

A muscular tube approximately 10 inches long, the esophagus is composed of four layers (external to internal): the fibrous, muscular (longitudinal and circular), submucous, and mucous coats. The distal end of the esophagus joins the proximal stomach at the gastroesophageal sphincter. This sphincter relaxes during swallowing to allow the bolus of food to enter the stomach.

3. Function

The esophagus is primarily responsible for food passage, which is accomplished by involuntary muscle relaxation and contraction, or peristalsis. The esophagus has some mucous secretion that aids in the movement of the food bolus.

B. Stomach

1. Location

The stomach lies inferior to the diaphragm in the epigastric, umbilical, and left hypochondriac areas of the abdomen (Figure 1-1). Proximally, it joins the esophagus at the gastroesophageal sphincter; distally, it is connected to the duodenum by the pyloric valve.

2. Description

The stomach is composed of four areas: the cardiac portion, the superior aspect that surrounds the gastroesophageal sphincter; the fundus; the body; and the pylorus, which joins the duodenum. The medial, concave side of the stomach is called the lesser curvature and the lateral, convex side is known as the greater curvature.

The first gastric coat is the outer, serous layer, which is continuous with the peritoneum. At the greater curvature, the peritoneum extends inferiorly, covering the intestines, and is known as the greater omentum. At the lesser curvature, it extends superiorly to the liver and is called the lesser omentum.

The second gastric coat is the muscular layer, composed of longitudinal, circular, and oblique muscles. This muscular arrangement breaks, churns, and mixes the food bolus.

The third, or submucous, coat consists of connective tissue.

The fourth, innermost layer (the mucous membrane) is arranged in folds, or rugae, that increase the surface area of the stomach and also house the secretory glands.

3. Function

The stomach has two primary functions: (1) mixing and transporting food and (2) secreting mucus and gastric fluids. Very little is absorbed in the stomach except for some water, salts, and weak acids such as alcohol and aspirin.

The gastric glands are named according to their location: The cardiac glands secrete mucin; the fundic glands secrete pepsinogen and acid; the pyloric glands secrete papsinogen and mucin. The mucous membrane cells produce gastrin. The stomach contents (chyme) empty into the duodenum when the intragastric pressure exceeds the intraduodenal pressure. The stomach is never completely empty, however, since mucin and gastric fluid are always present.

C. Small intestine

1. Location

The small intestine begins at the pyloric valve in the distal stomach and joins the large intestine at the ileocecal valve (Figure 1-1).

2. Description

The small intestine measures approximately 1 inch in diameter and consists of the duodenum (10 inches long), the jejunum (8 feet long), and the ileum (12 feet long). The four coats of the small intestine are the same as those of the stomach: an outer, serous layer; a muscular layer consisting of circular and longitudinal muscles; a submucous layer that contains Brunner's glands; and an inner layer, the mucous membrane, that houses the intestinal glands.

The circular fold arrangement and the presence of villi enlarge the surface area and thereby increase the potential for absorption. The ligament of Treitz is a suspensory ligament attached at the junction of the duodenum and the jejunum. It serves as an anatomic landmark.

3. Function

The small intestine is responsible for further digestion and absorption of chyme. It receives bile and pancreatic fluid to aid in the digestive process. The slow, weak peristaltic waves in this portion of gut facilitate digestion and absorption. The intestinal and Brunner's glands secrete intestinal fluids and mucus, respectively.

D. Large intestine

1. Location

The large intestine originates at the ileocecal valve and terminates at the rectum (Figure 1-1).

2. Description

The large intestine measures approximately 5 feet long and 2½ inches in diameter. The cecum, a blind pouch at the distal end of the small intestine below the ileocecal valve, measures approximately 2 to 3 inches in length. The appendix is suspended from the distal cecum.

The colon is divided into four segments. The ascending colon reaches to the underside of the liver, where it turns left at the hepatic flexure; it then becomes the transverse colon as it extends across the abdomen and reaches the lower edge of the spleen. At the splenic flexure, it runs downward to the iliac crest as the descending colon. The sigmoid colon begins at the level of the left iliac crest. The rectum, which measures approximately 7 to 8 inches long, leads into the anus, the final exit of the digestive tract.

The coats of the large intestine consist of the outer, serous layer, except in the rectum; the muscular layer; the submucous membrane; and the inner, mucous coat. (Unlike the corresponding small intestinal layer, this layer has no villi or circular folds.)

3. Function

The slow motility in the large intestine facilitates its primary function: the reabsorption of electrolytes and as much as 900 ml of water each day. The large intestine stores natural bowel flora; secretes mucus, potassium, and bicarbonate; and is responsible for defecation.

E. Pancreas

1. Location

The pancreas, situated behind the posterior curvature of the stomach (Figure 1-1), is divided into a head, a body, and a tail; the head is located within, and is attached to, the duodenal curve, while the tail stretches to the spleen.

2. Description

A gland approximately 6 inches long and 1 inch wide, the pancreas consists of connected lobes formed by groups of clustered cells (lobules). In each lobule is a branch of the pancreatic duct, or duct of Wirsung. The pancreatic duct runs from the tail to the head of the gland (Figure 1-2). This duct unites with the common bile duct from the gallbladder to form the ampulla of Vater, which empties into the duodenum.

The two types of cells that form the pancreas are the acinar cells and the beta cells of the islets of Langerhans. The acinar cells contribute to the exocrine functions of the pancreas, and the beta cells are responsible for its endocrine functions, notably the secretion of insulin.

3. Function

The pancreas, as noted, performs both endocrine and exocrine functions. The acinar cells secrete pancreatic fluid necessary for the digestive process in the small intestine; this fluid consists of digestive enzymes, water, and salt. Vagal stimulation causes the release of pancreatic fluid, along with the bicarbonate released by the duct-lining cells, from the pancreas through the pancreatic duct.

Figure 1-2 *Ductal system*

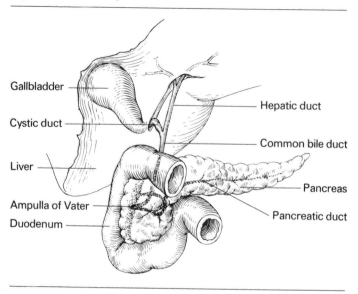

Gallbladder

Cystic duct

Liver

Ampulla of Vater

Duodenum

Hepatic duct

Common bile duct

Pancreas

Pancreatic duct

The islets of Langerhans, located close to the capillary system in the pancreas, perform the endocrine, or internal, function of the pancreas; they form and release insulin and glucagon into the bloodstream.

F. Liver

1. Location

The liver lies under the diaphragm in the right hypochondrium. It is also partly situated in the epigastrium of the abdomen (Figure 1-1).

2. Description

The liver is divided into two main lobes, the right and the left. The right lobe has two smaller lobes, the quadrate and the caudate. The liver has a connective tissue covering and also is partially covered by the peritoneum. The falciform ligament, a fold of the peritoneum, attaches the liver to the

Figure 1-3 *Venous drainage*

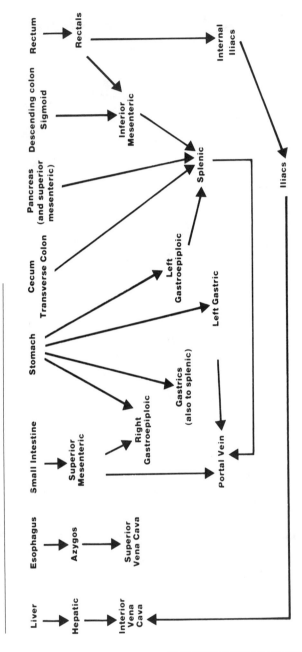

Figure 1-4 *Arterial blood supply*

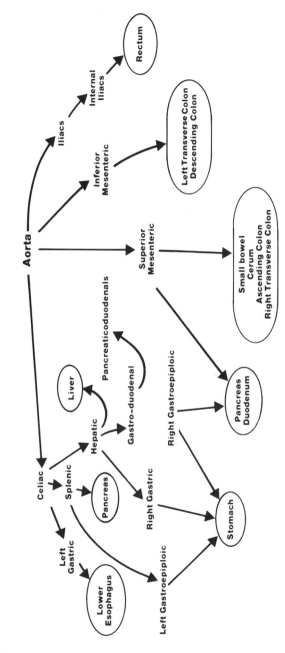

diaphragm and divides the right and left lobes. The round ligament secures the liver to the anterior abdominal wall at the umbilicus.

The lobes of the liver are composed of lobules (hepatic cells arranged in chains around a central vein), the working units of this organ. Sinusoids, through which blood flows, separate the hepatic chains. The sinusoids receive oxygenated blood from branches of the hepatic artery and nutrient-rich blood from branches of the hepatic portal vein (Figures 1-3 and 1-4). Kupffer cells line the sinusoids and are responsible for phagocytosis.

The hepatic cells remove oxygen, nutrients, and various poisons from the blood. These cells may also release certain other products into the blood. This function depends on the body's needs.

Bile canaliculi, located between the hepatic cells, empty the bile received from those cells into small bile ducts; these ducts finally join to form the right and left hepatic ducts (Figure 1-2). The common hepatic duct results from the merger of the right and left ducts; the cystic duct from the gallbladder later joins this common hepatic duct to form the common bile duct.

As previously discussed, the common bile duct and the pancreatic duct together empty into the duodenum through the ampulla of Vater. A valve situated in the common bile duct, known as the sphincter of Oddi, regulates the passage of gallbladder and liver secretions from this duct into the small intestine.

3. Functions

The liver performs such valuable functions that the body cannot survive without it. It produces and secretes bile, heparin, albumin, fibrinogen, and prothrombin. It collects and stores vitamins (A, D, E, and K), nutrients, glycogen, copper, iron, and some poisons. The liver is responsible for glyconeogenesis, for the destruction of bacteria and old red blood cells, and for the breakdown of poisons or toxic waste products.

G. Gallbladder

1. Location

The gallbladder lies on the posterior surface of the liver.

2. Description

The gallbladder has three coats: an outer, serous layer that is continuous with the peritoneum; a middle, smooth muscle layer; and an inner, mucous membrane layer. The inner layer is arranged in rugae, which enable the gallbladder to increase in size.

As previously mentioned, the cystic duct from the gallbladder joins the hepatic duct to carry bile into the common bile duct (Figure 1-2) and eventually into the small intestine. The sphincter of Oddi regulates flow from the common bile duct.

3. Function

The gallbladder primarily concentrates, stores, and secretes bile; it also absorbs water and electrolytes.

H. Spleen

Although the spleen is not involved in the digestive process, knowledge of its characteristics and function is necessary to its clinical discussion later in the text (see Chapter 6).

1. Location

The spleen lies in the left hypochondrium below the diaphragm (Figure 1-1).

2. Description

The spleen, a 5-inch mass of lymphatic tissue, is covered by a fibroelastic, smooth muscle capsule. The peritoneum then covers the capsule.

The functional tissue of the spleen is made up of white and red pulp. Red pulp contains venous sinuses and chains of tissue; white pulp consists of lymphoid tissue that surrounds arteries at intervals and is known as splenic nodules. The splenic pulp accounts for 25 percent of the reticuloendothelial system.

Figure 1-5 *Autonomic nervous system*

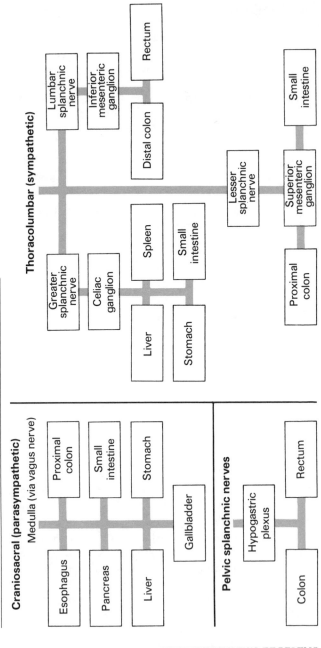

GASTROINTESTINAL PROBLEMS

3. Function

The spleen is responsible for phagocytizing old red blood cells, platelets, and bacteria, for manufacturing plasma cells and lymphocytes, and for storing and releasing blood. Contraction of the smooth muscle layer, produced by sympathetic stimulation (Figure 1-5), causes the release of stored blood from the spleen.

I. Innervation and blood supply

Figures 1-3 and 1-4 chart the arterial blood supply to and venous drainage from the gastrointestinal system. Figure 1-5 diagrams the sympathetic and parasympathetic innervation.

QUIZ

1. The three types of gastric glands are _____, _____, and _____.

2. Two gastric secretions are _____ and _____.

3. The _____ is a suspensory ligament that is attached to the junction of the duodenum and jejunum.

4. The greatest degrees of _____ and _____ take place in the small bowel.

5. In correct order, the four divisions of the colon are: _____, _____, _____, and _____.

6. The absorption of _____ and _____ takes place in the large intestine.

7. The endocrine secretions of the pancreas are

_____ and _____ ; the exocrine

secretion is _____.

8. True or false: The primary source of blood to the liver
is the portal system.

9. The common bile duct is formed by the union of the

_____ and the _____.

10. The bile that is formed and secreted by the _____

is stored and concentrated in the _____.

ANSWERS

1. Cardiac, fundic, pyloric.
2. Any of the following: pepsinogen/pepsin, hydrochloric acid, gastric acid, mucin.
3. Ligament of Treitz.
4. Digestion, absorption.
5. Ascending, transverse, descending, sigmoid.
6. Electrolytes, water.
7. Insulin, glucagon; pancreatic fluid.
8. True.
9. Cystic duct, hepatic duct.
10. Liver, gallbladder.

CHAPTER

History

OBJECTIVES

After completing this chapter, you will be able to:

1. Ask the questions necessary for a thorough gastrointestinal (GI) history

2. List the major elements of the GI history

3. List the three most frequent GI complaints.

A. Introduction

Many systemic diseases have GI manifestations; therefore it is essential to obtain a complete history when interviewing the patient. This chapter will cover those questions or aspects of the history that specifically relate to the GI system.

B. Conducting the interview

This chapter will not teach you how to conduct an interview, but the following recommendations should be kept in mind during the interviewing process.

1. Beginning

Begin the interview with a question like "How are you feeling?" or "What brought you here today?" Then follow the patient's lead.

2. Atmosphere

Promote an atmosphere of relaxed conversation, allowing the patient to speak freely rather than interrogating and overwhelming him or her with long lists of questions.

3. Questions

When you need more information on a specific topic, ask a leading question. Avoid questions that may be answered simply yes or no. Ask only one question at a time.

4. Terms

Use terms that the patient will understand, and be sure you understand all *his* terms. Don't proceed to the next question until you're sure that you and the patient have understood each other. Record the patient's answers in his own words.

5. Closing

At the end of the interview, summarize the information you have received and ask, "Is there anything I've missed?" or "Is there anything you'd like to add?"

C. Specific questions (Figure 2-1)

1. Age/sex/occupation

2. Present illness/chief complaint

a. Pain

- Location (localized versus generalized)
- Onset (when; slow versus rapid onset)
- Duration (how long has it been present; episodic versus continuous pain)
- Character (sharp, dull, tearing, cramping)
- Radiation
- Aggravating/precipitating factors
- Relief
- Times of occurrence
- Relationship to food, drugs, activity, position, bowel movements, breathing.

b. Nausea/vomiting

- Onset
- Duration
- Character (blood, bile, food products)
- Relief
- Times of occurrence
- Relationship to food, drugs, alcohol, activity, bowel movements
- Aggravating/precipitating factors
- Associated pain.

c. Bowel function

- Change in normal bowel habit
- Character of stool
- Constipation
- Diarrhea
- Frequency
- Excessive flatus
- Use of laxatives, enemas
- Rectal bleeding
- Relationship to food, drugs, alcohol

- Hemorrhoids
- Associated pain.

3. Weight

- Recent or significant gain
- Recent or significant loss
- No change
- Overweight or underweight according to standard height/weight proportion charts.

4. Diet

- Type of intake
- Appetite
- Change in eating or drinking habits
- Food intolerance
- Excessive belching.

5. Associated symptoms (GI and systemic)

- Chills
- Fever
- Indigestion
- Cold
- Flu
- Heartburn
- Dysphagia
- Distention.

6. Past medical history

- General health
- Illness (adult, childhood, psychiatric)
- Operations
- Injuries
- Hospital admissions
- Current medications
- Allergies
- Habits (smoking, drinking, drugs)
- Bleeding disorders
- Current treatments
- Menstrual history
- Exposure to infectious agents.

7. Family history (parents, grandparents, siblings)

- Ages
- General health/causes of death
- Specific diseases.

8. Psychosocial history

- Patient's description of his own emotional state (depressed, apathetic)
- Specific problems
- Stress
- Major changes in life-style.

D. Additional information

It may be helpful, even necessary in some cases, to obtain additional history information from sources other than the patient. Other sources include family members/significant others, previous hospital records, and family or other physicians.

Figure 2-1 *Patient assessment form*

Patient's name _____

Age _____ Sex _____ Occupation _____

Present illness or chief complaint _____

_____

Pain

Location _____

Onset _____

Duration _____

Character _____

Radiation _____

Aggravating/precipitating factors _____

_____

Relief _____

Time of occurrence _____

Relationship to food _____

            drugs _____

            activity _____

            position _____

            bowel movements _____

            breathing _____

Nausea/vomiting

Onset _____

Duration _____

Character _____

Relief _____

Time of occurrence _____

Relationship to food _____

            drugs _____

            alcohol _____

            activity _____

            bowel movements _____

Aggravating/precipitating factors _____

Associated pain _____

Bowel function

Change in normal habit _____

Character of stool _____

Constipation _____

Diarrhea _____

Frequency _____

Excessive flatus _____

Use of laxatives/enemas _____

Rectal bleeding _____

Relationship to food _____

drugs _____

alcohol _____

Hemorrhoids _____

Associated pain _____

Weight

Recent or significant gain _____

Recent or significant loss _____

No change _____

Overweight/underweight _____

Diet

Type of intake _____

Appetite _____

Change in habits _____

Food intolerance _____

Excessive belching _____

Associated symptoms (GI and systemic)

Chills _____   Heartburn _____

Fever _____   Dysphagia _____

Indigestion _____   Distention _____

Flu _____

Past medical history

General health _____

Illness (adult, childhood, psychiatric) _____

_____

Operations _____

Injuries _____

Hospital admissions _____

Current medications _____

Allergies _____

Habits (smoking, drinking, drugs) _____

Bleeding disorders _____

Current treatments _____

Menstrual history _____

Exposure to infectious agents _____

Family history (parents/grandparents/siblings)

Relationship   Age   General health/cause of death

_____   _____   _____

_____   _____   _____

_____   _____   _____

_____   _____   _____

_____   _____   _____

_____   _____   _____

_____   _____   _____

_____   _____   _____

_____   _____   _____

_____   _____   _____

Specific family diseases _____

_____

Psychosocial history

Emotional state _____

Specific problems _____

Stress _____

Major changes in life-style _____

QUIZ

1. List five major elements of the GI history:
2. List five components of the past medical history:
3. List the three most frequent GI complaints:
4. List four questions that help define pain:
5. List four questions that help define nausea/vomiting:
6. List three questions you should ask about the patient's diet:
7. Two sources for obtaining the patient's history (other than the patient) are _____ and

_____.

ANSWERS

1. Any of the following: age/sex/occupation, present illness, weight, diet, associated symptoms, past medical history, family history, psychosocial history.
2. Any of the following: general health, illness, operations, injuries, hospital admissions, current medications, allergies, habits, bleeding disorders, current treatments, menstrual history.
3. Pain, nausea/vomiting, and diarrhea.
4. Any of the following: location, onset, duration, character, radiation, aggravating/precipitating factors, relief, time of occurrence, relationship to food, drugs, position, activity, bowel movements, breathing.
5. Any of the following: onset; duration; character; relief; times of occurrence; relationship to food, alcohol, drugs, activity, bowel movements; aggravating/precipitating factors; associated pain.
6. Any of the following: type, appetite, change in habits, food intolerance, excessive belching. See Fig. 2-1 under subhead "Diet."
7. Any of the following: family member/significant other, old hospital records, other physicians.

CHAPTER

3

Assessment

OBJECTIVES

After completing this chapter, you will be able to:

1. *Identify the topographic segments used in the abdominal assessment and list the organs located in each*

2. *Examine the abdomen by inspection, auscultation, percussion, and palpation*

3. *Recognize normal and abnormal findings of the abdominal examination*

4. *Identify seven additional items that require assessment in the postoperative/post-trauma patient.*

A. Introduction

The GI assessment should be a systematic, thorough, four-step examination consisting of inspection, auscultation, percussion, and palpation; as you gain practice and experience, these four steps will intertwine with one another. If time is at a premium, as with the acutely ill or traumatized patient, this assessment must be performed rapidly: You can inspect the patient while you are auscultating, percussing, and so on. Although there is no need to keep them distinct during the assessment, this chapter presents the four steps separately.

B. Inspection

1. General appearance

As you first observe the patient, note his or her overall appearance, including facial expressions and body position (grimacing, thrashing, lying motionless).

2. Clothing

Remove all clothing to expose the entire abdomen while protecting the patient's privacy as much as possible. It is preferable to have the patient lie supine with arms at sides.

3. Architecture

Evaluate the abdomen for contour, shape, symmetry, and the presence of any visible masses. Figure 3-1 shows the abdominal quadrants and regions; note in which quadrant or region you find any abnormality.

4. Skin

Visually explore the skin for color, turgor, previous scars, lesions, herniations, superficial vessels, spider nevi, abnormal hair distribution, and ascites. In the trauma patient, look for local signs such as contusions, seat-belt burns (Figure 3-2), steering-wheel bruises, and ecchymotic areas (Cullen's and Grey Turner's signs). These findings provide clues about possible underlying organ injury.

If the patient has sustained a penetrating wound, look for entrance and exit sites. Leave penetrating objects in place until the patient is in a controlled environment and personnel qualified for object removal and patient after-care are in attendance.

5. Movement

Inspect and evaluate abdominal movement with respiration. Document any visible peristalsis or aortic pulsations.

Figure 3-1 *Abdominal quadrants (broken lines) and regions (solid lines)*

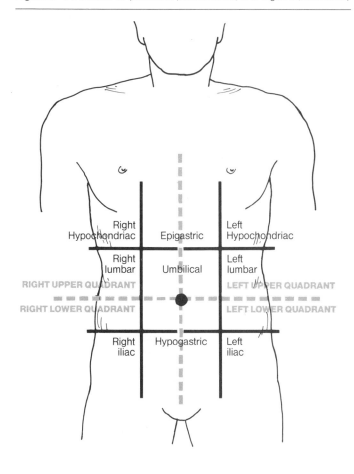

C. Auscultation

Auscultate the abdomen prior to percussion and palpation so as to avoid disturbing the bowel sounds. Begin auscultating in the right upper quadrant, lateral to the umbilicus, and proceed in a clockwise direction through all the quadrants (Figures 3-3 and 3-4). Evaluate the pitch, intensity, and frequency of the sounds. (Normal bowel sounds may be described as intermittent gurglings, swishings, or tinklings that are soft and high-pitched. They generally occur from 5 to 30 times per minute.)

Keep in mind that the presence of bowel sounds does not rule out intra-abdominal pathology and, conversely, the absence of bowel sounds is not always indicative of pathology. A finding more important than presence or absence of bowel sounds is absence of sounds in a patient who previously had normoactive sounds.

Figure 3-2   *Seat-belt burn*

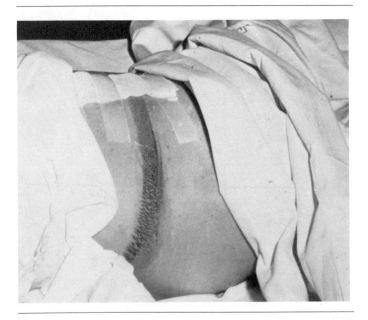

Figure 3-3 *Auscultation of right upper quadrant with diaphragm of stethoscope*

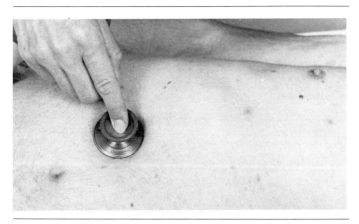

Listen also for friction rubs, which sound like two pieces of leather rubbing together. These sounds, usually heard over the liver or spleen, may signal hepatic/splenic irritation or rupture, an abscess, or peritoneal irritation.

Figure 3-4 *Auscultation of left upper quadrant with bell of stethoscope*

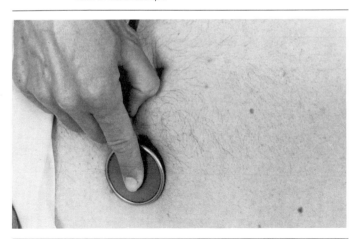

D. Percussion

Percuss the abdomen in a systematic fashion (as with auscultation) to locate abdominal viscera and help determine the approximate size of each organ (Figure 3-5). Gas-filled or hollow organs, such as the intestines and empty bladder (Figure 3-6), will emit tympanic or low-pitched sounds. Dense or solid organs (such as the liver and spleen), firm masses, or areas of fluid accumulation give off dull sounds when percussed. Muscles may be almost silent on percussion.

E. Palpation

1. Light palpation

With the palmar surfaces of the fingers, gently press approximately 1 cm deep in a systematic fashion through all quadrants (Figure 3-7). This light pressure helps relax the musculature of the abdomen and provides information about the general condition of the abdominal wall. Areas of pain and tenderness as well as superficial masses may also be identified. Any areas identified by the patient as painful should be palpated last, during deep palpation.

Figure 3-5 *Percussion of the abdomen*

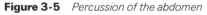
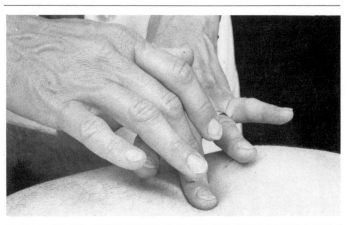

Figure 3-6 *Percussion of the bladder*

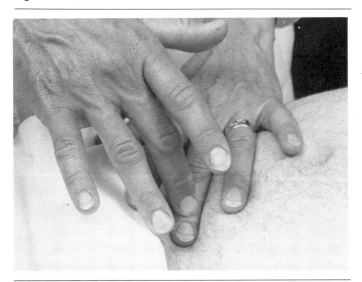

Figure 3-7 *Light palpation of the abdomen*

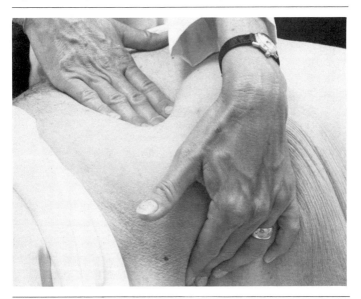

2. Deep palpation

During this phase of palpation, press your fingers to maximum depth (Figure 3-8). Instruct the patient to take slow, deep breaths to optimize relaxation. Deep palpation enables you to detect masses; the position, size, and any enlargement of organs; and the presence of rebound tenderness and/or referred pain. Evaluate all masses for position, size, consistency, shape, mobility, tenderness, and pulsation. Not all organs are normally palpable; usually, however, you can palpate the liver, splenic tip, cecum, sigmoid colon, and (occasionally) right kidney.

a. Spleen. To palpate the spleen, stand at the patient's left side. Place your right hand behind the costovertebral area parallel to the ribs and gently push upward. Work your left hand under the left costal margin (Figure 3-9). Have the patient take a deep breath. Since the spleen is pushed downward on inspiration, you should be able to palpate the tip.

Figure 3-8 *Deep palpation of the abdomen*

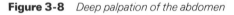

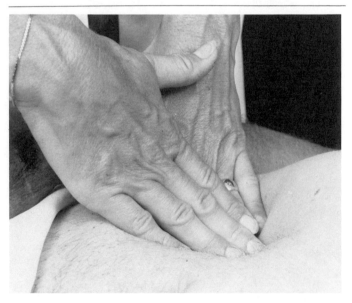

b. Liver. Palpate the liver in the same fashion as the spleen, but stand on the patient's right side and reverse the placement of your hands (Figure 3-10). On inspiration, the liver will be pushed down and you should be able to feel its lower edge tap against your fingers. The gallbladder lies behind the liver and will not be palpable unless it is enlarged or diseased.

Figure 3-9 *Palpation of the spleen*

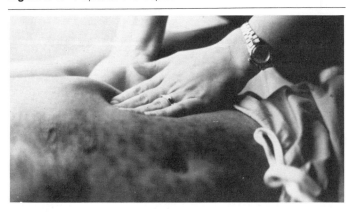

Figure 3-10 *Palpation of the liver*

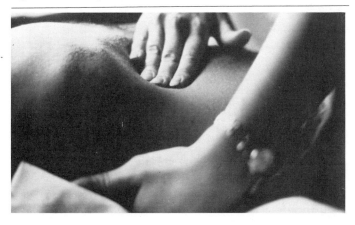

c. Kidneys/bladder. It usually is difficult to palpate the kidneys, especially the higher left kidney. To palpate, place one hand under the patient's flank and lift upward. Place your other hand on the midclavicular line at the level of the umbilicus and apply firm downward pressure. On inspiration, you may feel the lower pole of the kidney between the fingers of both hands. The empty bladder is not normally palpable (Figure 3-11). When full or distended, it will feel like a firm, smooth mass. An extremely distended bladder may easily be seen during the physical assessment.

Figure 3-11   *Palpation of the bladder*

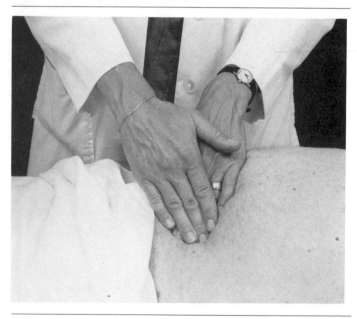

d. Hernias. Document any hernias that are visible or palpable (Figure 3-12) or that protrude when the patient coughs or strains. A reducible hernia is one in which the protuberance or hernial sac disappears when gentle pressure is applied to the site on a supine, relaxed patient. A hernia that will not reduce with pressure is called a strangulated or incarcerated hernia. Upon observing a hernia, note its location (incisional, inguinal, or umbilical) and whether it is reducible or nonreducible.

Figure 3-12 *Palpation for abdominal hernia*

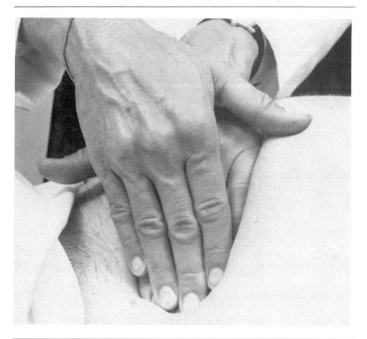

e. Back. Remember to assess the patient's back (Figure 3-13). This is especially important in the trauma patient and should be done as soon as he can be turned.

F. Recovery postoperative phase

To provide baseline information, perform the four-step abdominal exam on all emergency department or newly admitted patients and with every shift assessment. This systematic, often-repeated examination will enable you to

Figure 3-13 *Palpation of the back*

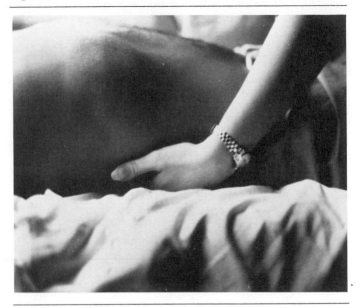

detect early changes or trends in the patient's condition. In the postoperative/post-trauma patient, you should also assess, monitor, and document (Figure 3-14) the following conditions/equipment:

1. Gastric/intestinal tubes (see Chapter 9)

- Correct placement
- Patency and functioning
- Proper method for securing the tube
- Drainage (consistency, color, odor, amount, gastric pH)
- Condition of nasal or oral mucosa.

2. Abdominal drains (see Chapter 9)

- Patency and functioning
- Proper method for securing the tube
- Drainage (consistency, color, odor, amount)
- Suction apparatus (proper degree of suction)
- Skin integrity around insertion sites.

3. Dressing

- Condition (dry, intact, saturated)
- Drainage on dressing (circle; note date and time).

4. Wounds/incisions

- Approximation of wound edges
- General skin condition around site
- Drainage from wound/incision
- Indications of inflammation/infection
- Integrity of any suture lines.

5. Alimentation

- Method of feeding (by mouth, enteral, parenteral)
- Type/amount
- Tolerance/residual
- Nausea/vomiting.

6. Elimination

- Passage of flatus/stools (amount, odor, color, con-
  sistency, frequency)
- Ostomies
- Impactions.

7. Medications

Patients with GI problems are likely to be receiving some
or all of the following:

- Antacids
- Antiemetics
- Cathartics
- Antispasmodics.

For each medication, document the dose, route, frequency,
and effectiveness.

Figure 3-14 *Postoperative patient assessment form*

Gastric/intestinal tubes

Check: _____ Placement

_____ Patency and functioning

_____ Method of securing

Describe drainage:

    Consistency _____

    Color _____

    Odor _____

    Amount _____

    Gastric pH _____

Describe condition of oral or nasal mucosa:

_____

Abdominal drains

Check: ____ Patency and functioning

    ____ Method of securing

    ____ Suction apparatus (proper degree of suction)

    ____ Skin integrity (around insertion sites)

Describe drainage:

    Consistency _____

    Color _____

    Odor _____

    Amount _____

Dressing

Check: ____ Condition (dry, intact, saturated)

    ____ Drainage on dressing (circle; note date, time)

Wounds/incisions

Check: ____ Approximation of wound edges

    ____ Condition of skin around site

    ____ Drainage from wound/incision

    ____ Indications of inflammation/infection

    ____ Integrity of any suture lines

Alimentation

Method of feeding: ____ Mouth

    ____ Enteral

    ____ Parenteral

Type/amount _____

Tolerance/residual _____

Nausea/vomiting _____

Elimination

Passage of flatus/stools:

      Amount _____

      Odor _____

      Color _____

      Consistency _____

      Frequency _____

Ostomies _____

Impactions _____

Medications _____

	Dosage	Route	Frequency	Effectiveness
Antacids				
Antiemetics				
Cathartics				
Antispasmodics				

QUIZ

1. Match the organ with the appropriate quadrant.

    Right upper _____ **a.** sigmoid colon

    Right lower _____ **b.** stomach

    Left upper _____ **c.** ascending colon

    Left lower _____ **d.** head of pancreas

2. Proper abdominal examination consists of the following four steps (in the correct order): _____,

_____, _____, _____.

3. True or false: Any penetrating objects in the abdomen should be removed immediately upon discovery.

4. True or false: The presence of bowel sounds indicates there is no pathology in the abdomen.

5. True or false: Palpation tells you whether an organ is solid or hollow.

6. True or false: It is difficult to palpate the left kidney even in healthy persons.

7. A hernia that will disappear with applied pressure is called _____.

8. List four additional items that should be included in your examination of the postoperative patient:

_____, _____, _____,

_____.

ANSWERS

1. Right upper _d._____
   Right lower _c._____
   Left upper _b._____
   Left lower _a._____

 2. Inspection, auscultation, percussion, palpation.

 3. False. A physician or other personnel qualified for aftercare must be present.

4. False. Bowel sounds may be normal even with intra-abdominal injury.

5. False. Percussion tells whether an organ is solid or hollow.

6. True.

7. Reducible.

8. Any of the following: drains, tubes, dressings, wounds, medications, alimentation, elimination.

C H A P T E R

Nausea/Vomiting/
Diarrhea

OBJECTIVES

After completing this chapter, you will be able to:

1. *Describe the nausea-retching-vomiting cycle and the symptoms for each phase*

2. *List three elements of treatment for nausea/vomiting and diarrhea*

3. *List three nursing considerations for the patient with nausea/vomiting and/or diarrhea.*

A. Nausea/vomiting

1. Nausea-retching-vomiting cycle

a. Nausea. Nausea, a psychic experience for which there is no specific definition, may be caused by many things, including pregnancy, pain, and motion. The phenomenon of nausea may or may not precede vomiting; it's associated with an autonomic discharge causing tachycardia, increased salivation, and perspiration. During the nausea phase of this cycle, the stomach is relaxed and its peristalsis slows; duodenal tone is increased.

b. Retching. Retching is the second phase of the cycle; during retching the pylorus contracts and the cardiac sphincter relaxes.

c. Vomiting. Vomiting is the ejection of gastric contents through the mouth. During this phase of the cycle, the pylorus is contracted, the cardiac sphincter rises and opens, and the gastric contents are expelled by increased pressure in the abdomen.

For this discussion of GI problems, nausea/vomiting will be considered as a single entity; its cause, treatment, and so on will be addressed accordingly.

2. Etiology

The symptom of nausea/vomiting is frequently reported and is associated with a large number of conditions. Many systemic diseases have associated GI symptoms, especially nausea/vomiting. Table 4-1 shows common causes/precipitating factors for nausea/vomiting.

3. Assessment

Immediately before vomiting, the patient will be tachycardic, dizzy or lightheaded, and weak. During the act of vomiting, the heart rate drops and the patient, who becomes pale, may complain of increased salivation and perspiration. Very often the patient will have to defecate at the same time. Assess the vomitus for character, quantity, odor, and color.

TABLE 4-1

PRECIPITATING FACTORS AND/OR
CAUSES OF NAUSEA/VOMITING

Psychogenic factors

Neurologic processes (meningitis, elevated intracranial pressure, head injury, space-occupying lesion)

Migraine headache

Systemic disease (organ failure, uremia)

Gastroenteritis (alcohol, virus, poisons, bacteria)

Gastric or intestinal obstructions

Cholecystitis

Appendicitis

Pancreatitis

Peptic ulcer disease

Pregnancy

Drugs/toxic agents—mercury, copper, alcohol, aspirin, histamine, meperidine hydrochloride (Demerol), antibiotics, etc.

Motion sickness

Anesthesia

Addisonian crisis

Radiation therapy

---

4. Diagnosis

Nausea/vomiting can be a symptom of a relatively minor condition (such as the "flu") or an early sign of an abdominal emergency (such as appendicitis). Diagnostic procedures are performed to help determine the cause of the nausea/vomiting and to evaluate its effect on the patient—for example, the degree of dehydration.

a. Patient history. The patient history is a most valuable diagnostic tool and, in some cases, may be sufficient to diagnose the cause of the nausea/vomiting.

b. Laboratory studies. Lab studies, such as electrolytes and chemical screening, will help evaluate the degree of dehydration. Complete blood count (CBC), amylase, enzymes, toxicology screens, and urinalysis will aid in diagnosing the cause of the nausea/vomiting.

c. Roentgenograms. Abdominal and chest films, barium studies, and cholecystograms may help in determining the cause of the nausea/vomiting.

d. Miscellaneous. Gastric aspiration, ECG, and ultrasound examination may be used as well.

5. Treatment

Early recognition of the cause of the nausea/vomiting is essential, for treatment must be aimed not only at the symptom and its effect on the patient, but also at its cause.

a. Gastric suction. Gastric suction will remove gastric contents and prevent potential aspiration into the lungs.

b. Medication. Antiemetics may be given when the nausea/vomiting is persistent and/or excessive. If a particular antibiotic or analgesic is the suspected cause, the drug (or its dosage) may need to be altered or discontinued. Post-traumatic or postoperative pain may cause nausea/vomiting; analgesia, while decreasing the pain, may also stop the nausea/vomiting.

c. Hydration. Volume replacement will be necessary if the patient has become dehydrated as a result of the nausea/vomiting.

d. Electrolytes. Electrolyte/acid-base disturbances must be corrected.

e. Cause. Treating the cause of the nausea/vomiting is most important. Surgical intervention may be necessary if the nausea/vomiting is related to a surgical abdominal problem (appendicitis, cholecystitis). Prophylactic measures, such as medication, may be instituted if the nausea/vomiting is related to pregnancy, radiation therapy, motion sickness, and so on. Psychiatric evaluation may be appropriate when psychogenic causes are suspected. Dietary changes may be required if the cause is a specific food intolerance.

6. Nursing considerations

a. Patient history/assessment. A thorough, total patient history and physical assessment are essential. (See Chapter 2 for specific information to be obtained concerning the nausea/vomiting pattern, diet, past medical history, psycho-social history, weight, and associated symptoms.)

b. Evaluate vomitus. Evaluate and document the character, color, and odor of the vomitus. Record and report findings such as blood, clots, and "coffee grounds." Test the vomitus for occult blood and pH. Measure and record the quantity of the vomitus and document the frequency of vomiting episodes.

c. Hydration. Assist with volume replacement. Closely monitor and record intake and output (including stools and gastric contents) and follow and report results of lab studies to evaluate hydration efforts.

d. Medication. Administer antiemetics, analgesics, sedatives, and so on. Monitor and record their degree of effectiveness.

e. Gastric suction. Maintain patency and proper functioning of gastric tubes to assure removal of gastric contents and prevent aspiration.

f. Patient preparation. Provide physical and psychological preparation and support prior to and during diagnostic studies as appropriate (see Chapter 11).

g. Complications. Be familiar with the types of patients likely to be at risk, as well as with the symptomatology, preventive measures, and treatment of the potential complications of nausea/vomiting. These complications include aspiration pneumonia, dehydration, electrolyte and acid-base imbalances (decreased potassium, decreased sodium, and alkalosis), and Mallory-Weiss syndrome (mucosal tear).

B. Diarrhea

Diarrhea may be defined as an increase in the amount, frequency, and/or fluidity of stools.

1. Etiology

Diarrhea may be caused by many factors and/or diseases, as shown in Table 4-2. Any single mechanism or a combina-

TABLE 4-2

CAUSES OF DIARRHEA

Malabsorption
Inflammatory bowel disease
Infections (bacteria, parasites)
Intestinal secretion disorders
Metabolic diseases (diabetes, hyperthyroidism)
Drugs (laxatives, antacids, antibiotics; see Table 4-4)
Fecal impactions
Partial bowel obstruction
Neoplasms
Functional bowel disease

tion may be active in the same patient. Four mechanisms that can cause diarrhea are:
- Altered intestinal motility
- Altered intestinal absorption
- Increased mucosal or vascular permeability in the bowel
- Presence of nonabsorbable, osmotically active solutes.

2. Assessment

a. Dehydration. Assess the patient with prolonged or excessive diarrhea for dehydration. Look at the vital signs; expect some degree of tachycardia and postural hypotension. The patient will probably be lethargic and weak. It is common to find poor skin turgor and mucosal dryness.

b. Pain. The patient may describe abdominal cramping and generalized abdominal tenderness.

c. Miscellaneous. Depending on the cause of the diarrhea, the patient may have nausea/vomiting and a fever. Bowel sounds are usually hyperactive.

3. Diagnosis

It is important to determine the cause of the diarrhea; often, however, it is more important to treat the sequelae of excessive or prolonged diarrhea — for example, dehydration — first. The diagnostic tools for diarrhea include:

a. History and physical assessment. The information obtained from a thorough patient history and physical assessment is often sufficient to diagnose the cause of diarrhea. The patient's description of the stool and the location and quality of any associated pain usually will suggest the cause (see Table 4-3).

b. Laboratory data. Lab studies (electrolytes, CBC, creatinine, BUN, and toxicology screens) may be ordered as appropriate.

c. Proctosigmoidoscopy. Proctosigmoidoscopy — visualization of the rectum and sigmoid colon — may be performed to identify the cause of the diarrhea. A proctosigmoidoscope is inserted into the rectum and sigmoid colon and the mucosa is examined for ulceration, polyps, friability, tumors, abscesses, and other pathologic signs. Mucosal smears and stool specimens may be obtained safely and easily during this study. Chapter 11 describes the nursing implications related to this procedure.

TABLE 4-3

CHARACTERISTICS OF DIARRHEA AND THEIR PROBABLE CAUSES

Characteristic	*Probable cause*
Bloody	Hemorrhage from lower GI tract
	Infection
	Inflammation
	Neoplasm
Bloody streaks	Hemorrhoids
	Fissure
Flecks of blood	Regional ileitis/colitis
	Meckel's diverticulum
Tarry appearance/melena	Digested blood from upper GI tract
Pus/exudate	Inflammation
	Infection
Pale, pasty, clay-colored	Biliary tract obstruction
Foamy, foul-smelling	Malabsorption
Nonbloody mucus	Irritable colon disease
Constipation alternating with diarrhea	Irritable colon disease
Painful diarrhea	Anal problem (fissure, perirectal abscess, tender hemorrhoid)

d. Roentgenograms. Abdominal films may be helpful in diagnosing ileus, obstruction, or calcification. Barium contrast studies (Chapter 11) may be ordered if a neoplasm or inflammatory bowel disease is suspected.

e. Stool specimen. The stool will be examined for parasites, fat, and gross or occult blood (guaiac test). If a bacterial cause of the diarrhea is suspected, a sample will be sent for cultures and gram stain.

4. Treatment

Treatment is usually directed at the causative or precipitating factor. Excessive or persistent diarrhea may require the use of medications such as kaolin and pectin (Kaopectate), diphenoxylate hydrochloride and atropine (Lomotil), and opiates. The last two agents decrease intestinal motility. The potential complications of prolonged, severe diarrhea (dehydration, acid-base disturbances, and sodium and potassium depletion) will require treatment as well, including electrolyte replacement and volume expansion.

5. Nursing considerations

a. Patient history. A thorough patient history is required, with emphasis on the diarrhea pattern (onset, duration, frequency, etc.); the relationship to food, drugs (see Table 4-4), and so on; associated symptoms; past medical history; psychosocial history; diet; and weight.

TABLE 4-4

ANTIBIOTICS ASSOCIATED WITH DIARRHEA

Ampicillin (Amcill, Omnipen, Polycillin, others)
Cephalexin (Keflex)
Cephalothin (Keflin)
Chloramphenicol (Chloromycetin)
Clindamycin (Cleocin)
Erythromycin
Lincomycin (Lincocin)
Neomycin
Penicillins
Tetracyclines

b. Evaluate stool. Check the patient for a fecal impaction if indicated. Evaluate a stool specimen for color, odor, and consistency. Record and report the presence of blood (gross and occult), mucus, pus, and/or undigested food particles. Send a stool sample for laboratory analysis if ordered. Measure and record the quantity of stools and document their frequency. In severe cases, it may be necessary to obtain a physician's order to insert a rectal tube in order to control output and prevent skin breakdown.

c. Hydration. Assist with volume replacement. Closely monitor and record intake and output (including stools) and follow and report the results of laboratory studies to evaluate hydration efforts.

d. Patient preparation. Provide physical and psychological preparation prior to diagnostic studies as appropriate (see Chapter 11).

QUIZ

1. _____ and _____ are two signs/symptoms of the prevomiting phase.

2. Three complications of nausea/vomiting include

   _____ , _____ ,

   and _____ .

3. The_____ is a valuable diagnostic tool for nausea/vomiting and diarrhea.

4. Evaluate vomitus and/or diarrhea for _____ ,

   _____ , _____ , and

   _____ .

5. Three signs/symptoms that indicate possible dehydration are _____ ,

   _____ , and _____ .

6. Two mechanisms responsible for producing diarrhea are increased intestinal _____ and decreased intestinal _____ .

7. True or false: If a patient is having diarrhea, you should check for a fecal impaction.

8. Two possible results of severe diarrhea are _____ _____ and _____ .

ANSWERS

1. Any of the following: tachycardia, dizziness/lightheadedness, increased salivation, weakness.

2. Any of the following: dehydration, Mallory-Weiss syndrome, aspiration pneumonia, electrolyte imbalance, acid-base disturbance.

3. Patient history.

4. Consistency, color, odor, amount.

5. Any of the following: tachycardia, postural hypotension, weakness, lethargy, poor skin turgor, dry mucosa.

6. Motility; absorption.

7. True.

8. Any of the following: potassium depletion, sodium depletion, dehydration, acid-base disturbances.

CHAPTER

5

Gastrointestinal Bleeding

OBJECTIVES

After completing this chapter, you will be able to:

1. Identify patients at risk for esophageal varices and peptic ulcer disease

2. List common symptoms of peptic ulcer disease and esophageal varices

3. List three nursing considerations for peptic ulcer disease and esophageal varices.

A. Introduction

An episode of gastrointestinal bleeding is considered a medical emergency, but it becomes a surgical emergency when the bleeding cannot be adequately controlled. This chapter will discuss general GI bleeding and also focus on peptic ulcer disease as well as esophageal varices.

B. Statistics

1. General GI bleeding

a. Etiology. The many diseases or causative factors that may precipitate GI bleeding are listed in Table 5-1.

b. Incidence. GI bleeding is one of the most common causes of emergency hospitalization and is associated with a significantly high mortality rate.

2. Peptic ulcer disease

a. Etiology. Peptic ulcers are erosions of the mucous membrane resulting from an excessive secretion of hydrochloric acid in relation to neutralization processes. (See Table 5-2 for the many causative or precipitating factors of peptic ulcer disease.)

TABLE 5-1

FACTORS THAT MAY CAUSE GI BLEEDING

LGI bleeds	UGI bleeds
Colonic tumors	"Erosive" disease (acute/chronic ulcer)
Ulcerative colitis	Hiatal hernia
Diverticulitis	Carcinoma
Hemorrhoids	Varices
Fissures	Excessive/chronic drug intake: alcohol, aspirin, steroids, phenylbutazone (Butazolidin), indomethacin (Indocin), anticoagulants, etc.
	Mallory-Weiss syndrome (Chapter 6)
	Trauma

TABLE 5-2

FACTORS THAT MAY CAUSE PEPTIC ULCER DISEASE

Shock
Sepsis
Central nervous system trauma
Respiratory failure (hypoxia)
Multiple organ failure
Multiple trauma
Burns
Drugs: aspirin, steroids, phenylbutazone,
    indomethacin, anticoagulants, etc.
Excessive alcohol intake
Metabolic disturbances
Genetic factors
Excessive intake of caffeine: coffee, tea, cola,
    Smoking
Gastritis
Stressful environment

b. Incidence. Peptic ulcer disease is responsible for approximately 50 to 70 percent of bleeding episodes. Peptic ulcer disease is most common in men 25 to 40 years of age, but it may affect people of either sex and any age. Ulcerations (often multiple lesions) may develop in the esophagus, stomach, pylorus, or duodenum. Duodenal ulcers occur 10 times more often than gastric ulcers.

3. Esophageal varices

a. Etiology. Esophageal varices (dilated, tortuous esophageal veins) result from increased pressure and resistance in the portal vein system. When hypertension occurs in the portal system, collateral circulation develops to compensate. Varices in the submucosa of the esophagus have no valve system; they are fragile and bleed easily. They may rupture as a result of vomiting, a Valsalva maneuver, or a gradual increase in portal pressure.

b. Incidence. Bleeding from esophageal varices accounts for approximately 17.5 percent of upper GI bleeding episodes and is most commonly seen in the cirrhotic patient.

C. Assessment

Table 5-3 shows the symptomatology of general GI bleeding, additional symptoms specific for peptic ulcers and bleeding esophageal varices, and symptoms indicative of hemorrhaging or perforated ulcers.

D. Laboratory studies

1. Baseline

Obtain baseline laboratory studies (CBC, coagulation, BUN, creatinine, electrolytes) on any patient with GI bleeding. Results commonly seen include decreased hematocrit/ hemoglobin levels, elevated WBC, coagulopathy, elevated BUN, and electrolyte imbalance.

2. Liver function

Obtain liver function studies as well, since patients with esophageal varices usually also have decreased liver function. Abnormal liver studies include elevated SGOT, SGPT, LDH, alkaline phosphatase, and bilirubin (direct and indirect).

E. Diagnosis

The patient history, clinical picture, and laboratory studies usually provide enough evidence to diagnose GI bleeding. Determination of the exact location or source of bleeding is important; however, measures to resuscitate the patient and stabilize his condition take precedence After the patient is hemodynamically stabilized, the following diagnostic studies or procedures may help locate the site of bleeding:

1. Insertion of Salem sump

A Salem sump (usually placed during resuscitation) may help to determine whether there is fresh blood in the stomach and therefore may identify the bleeding as upper GI (UGI, or above the ligament of Treitz).

2. Endoscopy

Endoscopy should be performed after the patient is stabilized, as rapid bleeding hinders accurate visualization. Further

TABLE 5-3

SYMPTOMS OF POTENTIAL GI BLEEDING

General	Peptic ulcer disease*	Esophageal varices
Emesis	Pain/discomfort	General symptoms
Hematemesis	Right/left upper	Hematemesis
Coffee grounds	quadrant	Melena
Feces	Midepigastric	Delirium tremens
Melena	Radiates through to	history
Hematochezia	back	Shock
Temperature	Lasts several days,	Hepatic encepha-
(low-grade for	then pain-free	lopathy
several days)	intervals	Jaundice
Hemodynamics	Worse with empty	Portal hypertension
Mild to moderate	stomach (before	causing:
Syncope	lunch, dinner,	Ascites
Orthostatic hypo-	bedtime)	Enlarged liver/spleen
tension	Wakes patient up	Spider nevi
Fatigue/weakness	at night	Anemia
Confusion	Relieved by food,	Palmar muscle
Severe to profound	milk, antacids	atrophy
Hypotension	Heartburn	Hemorrhoids
Tachycardia	Cramping/spasm	
Decreased urine	Fullness/pressure	
output	Anorexia	
Decreased cardiac	Reflex vomiting	
output	with or after	
Pallor	evening meal	
Thirst	Complications	
Diaphoresis	*Hemorrhage* (in 15-25% of ulcer patients)	
Anxious	Melena	
Stupor/coma	Blood in gastric tube, gross or guaiac-positive	
	Shock	
	(diaphoresis, tachycardia, hypotension)	
	Perforation	
	(highest incidence in middle-age group)	
	Acute, sudden abdominal pain	
	Referred pain (shoulder)	
	Increasing pain with movement	
	Vomiting	
	Distended, rigid abdomen	
	Peritonitis	
	Sepsis	
	Shock	

*In addition to general symptoms of GI bleeding.

treatment plans are usually decided upon after endoscopy identifies the bleeding source/site.

3. Sigmoidoscopy/colonoscopy

These procedures, performed 12 to 24 hours after excessive bleeding has stopped, are helpful in differentiating lower GI (LGI, or below the ligament of Treitz) from UGI bleeding.

F. Treatment

1. Hemodynamic resuscitation

Whatever the cause or source of GI bleeding, the primary goal of initial treatment is resuscitation and stabilization of the patient's hemodynamic status. The following measures should be taken:

- Insert large-bore intravenous catheters
- Replace fluids
- Closely monitor vital signs (Swan-Ganz triple-lumen catheter helps evaluate effects of resuscitation)
- Closely monitor laboratory studies
- Maintain adequate urine output
- Closely monitor intake/output (I/O) balance
- Closely monitor rate and amount of blood loss
- Replace blood and clotting factors
- Supplement O_2 as needed
- Obtain baseline chest roentgenogram and ECG
- Type and cross-match for sufficient packed red cells.

2. Peptic ulcer disease

a. Prevention. Steps to prevent peptic ulcer formation in high-risk patients are most important. Prophylactic measures would include:

- Control of gastric pH
- Use of antacids
- Administration of cimetidine
- Use of therapeutic diet and/or tube feeding.

b. Treatment. If GI bleeding due to a peptic ulcer occurs, the measures outlined under "Hemodynamic resuscitation," above, should be taken. In addition, the following may be appropriate:

- Gastric intubation/suction
- Gastric iced lavage (promotes vasoconstriction, removes clots, prevents aspiration)
- Sedation
- Antacids (neutralize acid, which causes pain)
- Norepinephrine administered down gastric tube
- Vasopressin administered IV.

When these measures cannot control bleeding, surgery may be required. It often includes:

- Vagotomy
- Oversewing or excision of ulceration
- More extensive removal/anastomosis.

3. Bleeding esophageal varices

Here again, resuscitation and treatment of hypovolemic shock are the first priorities. (See "Hemodynamic resuscitation," above.) Additional measures would include the following:

- Balloon tamponade (Sengstaken-Blakemore tube; see Chapter 9)
- Early intravenous or intra-arterial vasopressin (decreases mesenteric blood flow, which decreases portal hypertension)
- Steps to improve liver function
- Administration of vitamin K^+
- Administration of clotting factors and blood transfusions.

Postemergency measures should include plans for long-term alleviation of portal hypertension (shunting blood away from the portal system).

4. Angiography

When bleeding exceeds 0.5 ml/minute, angiography is generally required in all patients except those with esophageal varices. This procedure:

- Permits visualization of arterial and capillary systems
- Allows for the direct injection of vasopressors.

G. Nursing considerations

1. Patients at risk

It's vitally important to recognize and monitor all patients at risk for GI bleeding. Test emesis and stool for obvious and/or occult blood every 8 hours, record the results, and report any untoward findings. Likewise, record vital signs and laboratory data, and report any sudden changes or ominous trends.

2. Prophylactic measures

Specific nursing measures include the following:
- Monitor and record gastric pH every 2 to 4 hours; report a pH of less than 5.0
- Maintain patency and proper functioning of gastric decompression tubes (see Chapter 9)
- Administer antacids and titrate doses to maintain optimal pH
- Administer tube feedings as ordered, both as an acid buffer and for nutrition
- Focus patient teaching on behavior modification, including avoidance of smoking and excessive intake of alcohol, caffeine, drugs, and exposure to stress; offer instruction in proper nutrition and good eating habits.

3. Resuscitation

Assist with resuscitation efforts; closely monitor/document vital signs, laboratory data, and blood loss to evaluate effects of resuscitation.

4. Fluids

Closely monitor I/O (including gastric drainage/bleeding); be aware that urine output may decrease as a result of vasopressor drug action.

5. Vasopressin

Administer vasopressin (Pitressin) (see Chapter 10) as ordered. Be aware of potential side effects: bradycardia, hyponatremia, decreased cardiac output, decreased urine output, potential for cerebral and cardiac ischemia, myocardial infarction, abdominal colic/discomfort, and decrease in liver function.

6. Iced lavage

Monitor patient closely during iced lavage for hypothermia and potential complications: aspiration, respiratory arrest due to hypothermia, and cardiac arrest due to myocardial infarction.

7. Sengstaken-Blakemore tube

See Chapter 9 for nursing responsibilities when a Sengstaken-Blakemore tube is used.

8. Blood replacement

Assure that sufficient units of packed red cells are readily available for transfusion; follow hospital protocols for transfusion of blood or coagulation factors.

9. Reassurance

Provide reassurance and offer the patient brief, but honest, explanations.

10. Patient preparation

Prepare the patient physically (consent signed, type and cross-match blood, etc.) and psychologically for surgery when appropriate.

QUIZ

1. The most common cause of GI bleeding is

_____ .

2. Burns, shock, and excessive alcohol intake are precipitating factors for _____ .

3. Esophageal varices result from increased

_____ and _____ in the

_____ .

4. The primary goals in initial treatment of a GI bleed are

_____ and _____.

5. The most immediately life-threatening complication of a GI bleed is _____.

6. Ascites, spider nevi, and enlargement of the liver and spleen are symptoms of _____.

7. True or false: Prevention is the best treatment for peptic ulcer disease.

8. True or false: The main purpose of a Sengstaken-Blakemore tube is to provide for iced gastric lavage.

ANSWERS

1. Peptic ulcer disease.
2. Peptic ulcer disease.
3. Pressure; resistance; portal vein system.
4. Resuscitation; stabilization.
5. Hypovolemic shock.
6. Portal hypertension.
7. True.
8. False. The Sengstaken-Blakemore tube provides balloon tamponade.

6

Trauma

OBJECTIVES

After completing this chapter, you will be able to:

1. *Describe two types of esophageal injuries*

2. *Recognize common symptoms of a perforated esophagus and specific intra-abdominal injuries*

3. *List six complications associated with abdominal trauma in the postoperative phase.*

A. Esophageal trauma

Esophageal injuries may result from internal trauma (as with Mallory-Weiss syndrome or an endoscopic accident) or from external trauma (either blunt or penetrating). Mallory-Weiss syndrome involves a laceration, usually longitudinal, that occurs at or near the gastroesophageal junction. The right posterior esophageal wall is the most common site. Since the esophagus is well protected, injury to this structure from external blunt trauma is seen less frequently than penetrating injury. Perforation of the esophagus during endoscopy, an iatrogenic injury, is probably the most common cause of esophageal injury.

1. Etiology

External trauma and endoscopic accidents are self-explanatory. Mallory-Weiss or mucosal lacerations occur most frequently as a result of forceful retching and vomiting. This tear occurs most often in men; excessive aspirin ingestion and alcohol abuse are the causative factors 20 percent and 40 percent of the time, respectively. This tear also occurs in patients with pre-existing hiatal hernias and is a frequent cause of UGI bleeding.

2. Assessment

a. Mallory-Weiss syndrome. Look for hematemesis, the most common symptom. The patient may also describe midepigastric pain that pierces through to the shoulder blades.

b. Perforation. The patient who sustains an esophageal injury from endoscopic perforation or external trauma usually develops subcutaneous air in the neck, face, and/or chest wall. Mediastinal air will be apparent on chest roentgenogram within several hours. Also assess the patient for:
- Shortness of breath
- Diaphoresis
- Cyanosis
- Pallor
- Tachycardia
- Fever (within 24 hours)

- Abdominal pain/tenderness
- Epigastric muscle spasms
- Mild to severe chest/midepigastric pain
- Shock.

3. Diagnosis

a. History. The patient's history will often suggest the diagnosis. The patient with Mallory-Weiss syndrome may report having eaten a heavy meal or having a pre-existing gastric disturbance that is followed by retching and vomiting (hematemesis) and then pain. A history of drug intake (aspirin, alcohol, etc.) will also be of value. The development of the previously mentioned symptoms after endoscopy should alert you to probable esophageal perforation.

b. Diagnostic studies. The following studies will serve to confirm the diagnosis suggested by the patient's history:
- Roentgenograms (upright chest studies with radio-paque or water-soluble contrast medium)
- Endoscopy
- Angiography
- Laboratory studies, including coagulation profile.

4. Treatment

The decision for either emergency surgery or simply supportive care will be made after the site of perforation and/or bleeding has been established.

a. Mallory-Weiss syndrome. Blood loss from these tears is usually small and self-limiting; therefore supportive care is usually the treatment of choice. Hemorrhage with arterial involvement, however, could possibly require vasopressin, clot embolization, tamponade, or surgery for ligation of bleeders and/or closure.

b. Perforations. Resuscitative measures may be required initially, followed by surgery to restore esophageal integrity. After surgery, drains and antibiotics are used to prevent infection.

5. Nursing considerations

- Obtain thorough patient history
- Assist with and monitor resuscitation efforts
- Assure patency and proper functioning of gastric tube
- Assure sterile management of drainage from operative site
- Monitor patient for signs of infection and hemorrhage.

Figure 3-14 shows a postoperative assessment form that may be helpful in the care of patients with esophageal trauma.

B. Abdominal trauma

1. Diagnostic problems

Intra-abdominal injuries may result from penetrating or blunt trauma; they are most often caused by vehicular accidents. Detecting and diagnosing intra-abdominal pathology is often difficult because the victim of blunt trauma frequently has associated injuries (as to the head or spinal cord) and/or may also suffer from drug or alcohol intoxication, which alters his level of consciousness and pain sensation. Penetrating injuries from gunshot or stab wounds can also be misleading, since it is impossible to determine the precise path of the missile or blade by visual, physical, or radiologic examinations.

2. Assessment and index of suspicion

Prompt detection and accurate diagnosis of an intra-abdominal injury may be accomplished by the use of three tools: repeated assessment, a high index of suspicion, and peritoneal lavage. Thorough, repeated abdominal examinations using the four basic steps (inspection, auscultation, percussion, and palpation), as described in Chapter 3, is essential in the detection of injury and/or significant changes and in monitoring trends in the patient's condition. Symptoms that should raise your suspicions concerning specific injuries will be highlighted under "Assessment," below. A good working knowledge of frequently seen symptoms is the basis for your index of suspicion, the second tool used in detecting and diagnosing intra-abdominal injury.

3. Peritoneal lavage

Peritoneal lavage, the third tool, can confirm the presence of intra-abdominal pathology. It is a quick, safe, accurate procedure performed during the early admission phase. Although lavage does not indicate which organ is damaged, it does reflect the severity of the injury and confirm or negate the need for an exploratory laparotomy. Actual diagnosis of specific organ injuries is then made during surgical exploration. (See Chapter 11 for a discussion of peritoneal lavage and the nurse's responsibilities during this procedure.)

4. Assessment

a. Spleen. The spleen is the organ most often injured by blunt abdominal trauma. The symptomatology, however, will be similar whether the mechanism of injury is blunt or penetrating trauma. Suspect a splenic injury in any patient who has sustained lower thoracic or upper abdominal trauma.

The patient may have:
- Local sign of injury (contusion, open wound)
- Abdominal tenderness, guarding
- Left upper quadrant pain
- Kehr's sign
- Left lower rib fractures
- Falling hemoglobin/hematocrit
- Elevated white blood cell count
- Elevated platelet count
- Shock
- Positive peritoneal lavage.

b. Liver. Of the abdominal organs injured by blunt trauma, the liver suffers the second highest number of injuries. Both penetrating and blunt mechanisms, however, create similar symptoms. Hepatic injury is to be suspected in any patient with upper abdominal or lower thoracic trauma.

The patient may have:
- Local sign of injury (contusion, open wound)
- Right upper quadrant pain
- Abdominal tenderness and guarding

- Hemorrhagic shock
- Falling hemoglobin/hematocrit
- Right rib fractures
- Increased pain on cough or deep breath
- Positive peritoneal lavage (possibly gross blood).

c. Small bowel. Injury to the small bowel may be caused by blunt or penetrating trauma. Symptoms may vary from no obvious sign of trauma to acute symptoms of peritoneal inflammation.

Assess the patient for:
- Right upper quadrant pain
- Pain radiating to shoulder, back, chest
- Nausea, vomiting
- Elevated white blood cell count
- Shock
- Positive peritoneal lavage.

d. Colon. Colonic injuries are most commonly due to penetrating trauma, specifically gunshot wounds. Injuries resulting from blunt trauma are not seen frequently; however, they are associated with improperly worn seat belts. Colonic injuries usually present with symptoms of peritonitis, since this portion of the bowel has a high bacterial count.

Look for:
- Local sign of injury (contusion, open wound)
- Nausea, vomiting
- Abdominal pain or tenderness
- Referred or rebound pain
- Absent bowel sounds
- Positive peritoneal lavage.

e. Duodenum. Duodenal injury rarely occurs as a result of blunt trauma but may be seen with crush injuries (steering wheel) or direct blows. Detection of such an injury may be difficult if the bleeding or leaking of duodenal contents occurs in the retroperitoneal space. There may be no acute clinical signs and the peritoneal lavage is usually negative. Peritoneal bleeding, however, will create symptoms of peritonitis. A duodenal injury frequently accompanies another intra-abdominal injury, specifically a pancreatic injury, resulting in a variety of symptoms.

Assess this patient for:
- Local sign of injury (contusion, open wound)
- Right upper quadrant pain, tenderness
- Referred pain to the shoulder, back, groin, or testicles
- Vomiting
- Elevated white blood cell count, serum amylase
- Positive peritoneal lavage.

f. Pancreas. Pancreatic injuries may result from penetrating or, more rarely, blunt trauma (crushing from a steering wheel). They are seen only occasionally as isolated injuries; when they do occur, it's frequently in conjunction with splenic injuries.

Detection of a pancreatic injury is difficult early after the injury, since clinical signs (such as epigastric pain and tenderness) may be delayed for several hours. A pancreatic injury is often detected when the patient is surgically explored for other suspected intra-abdominal pathology. Consider any patient with upper abdominal trauma, T_{11}-L_2 spine fractures, and/or elevated or rising serum amylase levels as possibly having pancreatic injuries.

g. Stomach. The empty stomach is rarely injured by blunt trauma as it is well protected and is a fairly mobile organ. Gastric injuries occur more frequently from penetrating trauma, specifically gunshot wounds. Since it is a hollow organ, the stomach, upon injury, will rupture and spill its contents. The patient with a gastric injury therefore may exhibit signs of peritoneal inflammation, such as generalized abdominal pain and tenderness.

The patient with a gastric injury frequently has a positive peritoneal lavage. Also suspect a gastric injury when the gastric tube reveals fresh or persistent bleeding. It is important to differentiate this blood from blood the patient may have swallowed secondary to maxillofacial injuries.

5. Nursing considerations

In the acute, preoperative phase, nursing responsibilities do not differ for specific organ injuries since diagnostic confirmation is not made until the patient has been surgically explored. Patient stabilization and preoperative preparation are the goals of nursing care regardless of the suspected intra-abdominal injury.

a. Volume expansion. After establishing several large-bore intravenous catheters, closely monitor volume expansion. Accurate I/O records are essential to monitor the adequacy of the resuscitation measures instituted.

b. Vital signs. Closely monitor and record vital signs (blood pressure, pulse, respiration, temperature) as well as central venous pressure. Common findings in the early, acute phase include tachycardia with hypotension. Report any significant changes or trends to the primary physician.

c. Blood replacement. Assure that the patient has been typed and cross-matched for 6 to 12 units of packed red cells and that the blood is available as soon as possible. The unstable patient may require transfusions to improve preoperative hemodynamic status. This often means that type-specific or un-cross-matched blood must be utilized.

Coagulopathy occasionally develops preoperatively, and the patient may require transfusions of clotting factors such as fresh frozen plasma or platelets. Communicate your specific needs to the blood bank as soon as possible. Follow hospital policies regarding transfusion of blood and blood by-products.

d. Assessment. Continued, close observation and assessment of the patient's overall status are necessary to detect change or downward trends. These include not only the hemodynamic factors but also repeated abdominal examinations. These measures are especially important when the decision to operate has not yet been made or if the physician chooses to monitor and observe the patient for a longer period of time. The nurse at the bedside is usually the first person to detect the change that may signal deterioration in the patient's condition.

e. Operative consent. Assist the physician, when appropriate, in obtaining the patient's consent for surgery. Many times the patient is unable to sign the consent for a variety of reasons, such as an altered level of consciousness or drug or alcohol intoxication. Follow state laws and hospital policies in these cases. Assist the physician when informing the family of operative procedures that are needed.

f. Baseline laboratory studies. The following studies are ordered for all patients with abdominal trauma:
- Hematocrit/hemoglobin
- WBC
- Platelet count
- PT/PTT
- Amylase
- Electrolytes.

If intra-abdominal injury is not positively confirmed by peritoneal lavage and the patient is stable, the physician may want to monitor the hematocrit/hemoglobin closely for a specific period of time. Frequently, hematocrit/hemoglobin readings are ordered every 4 hours. Be sure that all blood studies are sent as ordered and that results are reported to the physician.

g. Discretionary laboratory studies. The following tests may be ordered in addition to the baseline studies listed above:
- SGOT
- SGPT
- LDH
- Alkaline phosphatase
- Bilirubin — direct and indirect.

In addition, it is wise to obtain a hepatitis antigen-antibody level and toxicology screens for drug and alcohol levels.

h. Peritoneal lavage. Anticipate the need for a lavage in a patient with any of the following symptoms or associated

injuries (see Chapter 11 for a discussion of the peritoneal lavage procedure and nursing responsibilities):
- A history of blunt abdominal trauma
- Tender or painful abdomen
- Thoracic or lumbar spine fractures
- Pelvic fractures
- Alterations in consciousness or sensation.

C. Complications of acute abdominal trauma

1. Hemorrhage

a. Causes. Poor surgical hemostasis; continued bleeding from liver lacerations, splenic fractures, or hematomas; coagulation factor "washout" due to multiple transfusions.

b. Occurrence. Any time pre- or postoperatively.

c. Nursing implications. Observe for signs of shock and increasing abdominal girth; monitor I/O, including bloody drainage from wounds and drains. Monitor coagulation studies (PT, PTT, platelets, fibrinogen, and fibrin split products; platelet deficiencies are common after multiple transfusions). Apply MAST suit as indicated; screen patient for hepatitis Australian antigen titer; use caution when handling dressings, sump drainage, and banked blood products. Follow hospital protocols for transfusion of blood and clotting factors and autotransfusion. Explain procedures to patients when appropriate.

2. Abscess

Abscesses are usually subhepatic or subphrenic.

a. Causes. Traumatic contamination; faulty aseptic technique; inadequate drainage of dependent intra-abdominal spaces.

b. Occurrence. From 48 hours to weeks after trauma.

c. Nursing implications. Maintain drain patency; change drain suction apparatus daily to prevent retrograde contamination; monitor color, odor, and amount of drainage; use aseptic technique when handling drains and changing dressings. Position patient on alternate sides every 2 hours to prevent subphrenic fluid accumulation; observe for signs of subphrenic infection (hiccups due to diaphragmatic irritation, local tenderness in subcostal spaces, axillae, and shoulders) and subhepatic infection (right upper quadrant pain, abnormal liver function tests, nausea/vomiting, and fever).

3. Wound infection

a. Causes. Traumatic contamination; faulty aseptic technique; inadequate drainage of dependent intra-abdominal spaces.

b. Occurrence. Beginning 8 to 10 hours after trauma.

c. Nursing implications. Use strict aseptic technique when handling drains and dressings; monitor wound drainage, redness, warmth, and incision line separation; change dressings every 4 to 8 hours; dispose of contaminated dressings in separate plastic bag.

4. Dehiscence and evisceration

a. Causes. Poor or delayed wound healing; abdominal distention; increased intra-abdominal pressure.

b. Occurrence. Postoperatively.

c. Nursing implications. Sedate patient as ordered to prevent straining and restless movement. Ensure patency and proper functioning of gastric tubes and wound drains. Instruct patient to splint abdominal wounds with pillows when coughing or suctioning. Monitor incision line integrity. Report separation or sudden drainage from abdominal wound. If *dehiscence* occurs, apply abdominal binder to prevent progression. If *evisceration* occurs, cover viscera with gauze soaked in normal saline. With either dehiscence or evisceration, notify physician and prevent further movement of patient.

5. Primary peritonitis

a. Causes. Ascending colonization of female genital tract; nephrosis; cirrhosis; trauma; surgical contamination.

b. Occurrence. Any time after trauma or surgery.

c. Nursing implications. Observe for nausea and vomiting (usually the first signs), increased nasogastric drainage, decreased or absent bowel sounds, increased local or generalized pain, rebound tenderness, lack of movement or position changes. Monitor laboratory data, especially WBC and platelets. Monitor vital signs and temperature. Ensure patency and proper functioning of gastric tubes and drains. Administer pain medications and antibiotics as ordered. Monitor I/O, replacing fluids as ordered. Observe for signs of respiratory involvement (e.g., refusal to cough or breathe deeply).

6. Retroperitoneal hematoma

a. Causes. Blunt or penetrating abdominal trauma; pelvic fracture; disruption of retroperitoneal veins.

b. Occurrence. Immediately to several hours after trauma.

c. Nursing implications. Monitor vital signs frequently; monitor lab data, especially hemoglobin and hematocrit. Observe patient for abdominal rigidity, Grey Turner's sign, and local or generalized pain of the back, flank, or abdomen. Monitor urinary output for amount and hematuria.

7. Paralytic ileus

a. Causes. Excessive or rough handling of bowel during surgery; retroperitoneal hematoma; narcotic administration; premature removal of gastric tube; shock; sepsis; peritonitis.

b. Occurrence. Any time after trauma or surgery.

c. Nursing implications. Prevent by intestinal intubation; maintain patency and proper functioning of gastric tubes and drains (check every 2 hours). Auscultate abdomen for decreased or absent bowel sounds. Discontinue narcotics as soon as possible; monitor for complaints of extreme discomfort, cramps, or vomiting. Observe abdomen for distention and dehiscence.

8. Pancreatitis

a. Causes. Traumatic contusion; surgical manipulation; alcohol abuse.

b. Occurrence. From 2 hours to 2 days after trauma.

c. Nursing implications. Observe for severe midepigastric pain radiating to the back and unrelieved by high doses of narcotics, general abdominal pain and rigidity, paralytic ileus or abdominal distention, ascites, jaundice, vomiting, signs and symptoms of infection, assumption of knee-chest position. Auscultate breath sounds for indications of effusion or atelectasis. Monitor lab data for increased serum amylase, serum lipase (possibly delayed up to 120 hours), urinary amylase, hyperglycemia. Monitor patency and functioning of gastric tubes and drains. Administer analgesics as ordered (morphine will increase serum lipase and amylase levels); administer antibiotics as ordered; administer short-acting insulin as ordered. Position patient in semi-Fowler's position to increase lung expansion and prevent enzyme and fluid accumulation in the lungs.

9. Respiratory involvement

Common post-traumatic complications include pleural effusion, pneumonia, and atelectasis.

a. Causes. Surgical manipulation; decreased lung expansion due to pain; lowered level of consciousness; subdiaphragmatic fluid pressure.

b. Occurrence. Any time postoperatively.

c. Nursing implications. Turn and position the patient every 2 hours; administer chest physiotherapy every 4 to 6 hours; place patient in Fowler's position to prevent subphrenic fluid pooling (don't leave patient supine for prolonged periods). Auscultate breath sounds frequently; suction often if patient is intubated; encourage coughing and deep breathing exercises and use of incentive spirometer. Monitor patient for hiccups or being out of phase with ventilator (indicative of subphrenic abscess). Monitor arterial blood gas values and daily chest films.

QUIZ

1. The organ most frequently injured by blunt abdominal trauma is the _____.

2. List three symptoms of a hepatic injury:

   _____,

   _____,

   _____.

3. The pancreas is frequently injured in conjunction with the _____.

4. List five nursing considerations for the patient with an intra-abdominal injury: _____,

   _____, _____,

   _____, _____.

5. True or false: Peritoneal lavage should never be performed on an unconscious or intoxicated patient.

6. True or false: A patient with a severe liver injury may develop a coagulopathy preoperatively.

7. List five potential complications of abdominal trauma:

_____,

_____,

_____,

_____,

_____.

8. Hiccups due to diaphragmatic irritation may signal

_____.

9. A mucosal tear at or near the gastroesophageal junction is called a _____.

10. True or false: Esophageal injuries usually require only supportive care.

ANSWERS

1. Spleen.

2. Any of the following: local sign of injury, right upper quadrant pain, abdominal tenderness, guarding, hemorrhagic shock, falling hematocrit/hemoglobin, right rib fractures, increased pain on cough or deep breath, positive peritoneal lavage.

3. Spleen.

4. Any of the following: volume expansion, vital signs, blood therapy, assessment, operative consent, laboratory studies, peritoneal lavage.

5. False. Peritoneal lavage is indicated for any patient with altered level of consciousness or sensation because the physical examination may be inadequate.

6. True.

7. Any of the following: sepsis (wound infection, abscess), hemorrhage, paralytic ileus, coagulopathy, peritonitis, pancreatitis, pulmonary complications, dehiscence/evisceration.

8. A subphrenic abscess.

9. Mallory-Weiss syndrome.

10. False. Except for minor, self-limiting Mallory-Weiss lacerations, most esophageal injuries require surgery.

Nonsurgical Problems

OBJECTIVES

After completing this chapter, you will be able to:

1. State the two common causes of acute pancreatitis
2. List three symptoms of acute pancreatitis
3. Name the classic sign of paralytic ileus
4. List three nursing considerations for acute pancreatitis and for paralytic ileus.

A. Acute pancreatitis

Acute pancreatitis, or autodigestion of the gland by enzymes, may be hemorrhagic or nonhemorrhagic. It is a serious disease, and the significant mortality resulting from it is usually due to shock and other complications.

1. Etiology

Alcoholism and biliary tract disease are the most common causes of pancreatitis, accounting for approximately 80 percent of the cases. Table 7-1 lists many other causes or precipitating factors.

2. Assessment

The clinical picture you observe may present symptoms that range from mild to severe. The classic symptom in nearly all patients, however, is pain. Assess the patient for the following:

a. Pain. The pain described may be mild to excruciating. It is usually described as steady, sharp, twisting, or stabbing; in location, it is midepigastric and/or in the left upper quadrant, with a boring type of radiation to the back and/or flank. There may be generalized or rebound tenderness and guarding as well. The pain may develop in crescendo fashion or have an abrupt, severe onset. An attack frequently occurs after a large intake of food or alcohol, and the pain

TABLE 7-1

CAUSES OF PANCREATITIS

Alcoholism	Idiopathic causes
Biliary tract disease	Hypercalcemia
Trauma	Hereditary
Postoperative procedures	Peptic ulcer disease
Drugs	Metabolic disorders
Cancer	Infectious diseases
Pregnancy	

increases when the patient is lying supine. It usually lasts for several days and then gradually ceases. The patient may experience relief by fasting, maintaining the knee-chest position or leaning forward, or (frequently) vomiting. The pain of acute pancreatitis is not usually relieved by narcotics.

b. Nausea/vomiting. Nausea and vomiting are seen in most patients with acute pancreatitis.

c. Fever. A temperature $1°$ to $2°F$ above normal is a common symptom.

d. Ileus. Paralytic ileus (abdominal distention, tenderness, decreased bowel sounds) results from inflammation of the peritoneum. Fecal vomiting may occur if the ileus is severe.

e. Respiratory involvement. The patient with acute pancreatitis often has jerky, painful respirations and some degree of respiratory distress. An elevated diaphragm, atelectasis, infiltrates, and/or effusions are frequently seen on chest roentgenograms.

f. Jaundice. Mild jaundice — usually scleral yellowing — may be seen in approximately 20 percent of the patients.

g. Shock. Shock resulting from hemorrhage, hypovolemia, and protein loss to third spaces and the gut is seen in the more severe cases (Table 7-2).

TABLE 7-2

POTENTIAL COMPLICATIONS OF ACUTE PANCREATITIS

Time	Complication
Early	Shock
	GI bleeding
	Hypocalcemia
	Jaundice
Late	Pseudocyst
	Abscess
	Pancreatic ascites

h. Miscellaneous. Coagulation disorders, hypocalcemia, and ascites may be experienced in varying degrees. Cullen's or Grey Turner's signs, due to retroperitoneal pancreatic hemorrhage, may be observed. (see Table 7-2).

3. Laboratory studies

a. Amylase. Serum amylase levels, though not indicative only of pancreatitis, usually rise within 2 hours of the onset of the attack and remain elevated. They usually return to normal 3 to 4 days later. Urinary amylase levels rise earlier and usually remain elevated longer than do serum levels.

b. Lipase. Serum lipase levels parallel amylase levels but remain elevated longer. Lipase, however, is not indicative only of pancreatitis.

c. Complete blood count. Anemia may be seen. The WBC is usually 10,000 to 30,000, and the sedimentation rate is elevated.

d. Glucose. A transient hyperglycemia is usually seen.

4. Diagnosis

The patient's history, clinical picture, and laboratory studies, in some cases, may provide enough evidence to diagnose acute pancreatitis. Chest and abdominal roentgenograms, upper GI series, ultrasound exams, and CAT scans may also offer significant data. Oral or intravenous cholangiography may help with the differential diagnosis. Additional laboratory studies are indicated, including arterial blood gases (ABGs), enzymes (SGOT, LDH, alkaline phosphatase), calcium, magnesium, lipids, and bilirubin.

5. Treatment

Treatment of acute pancreatitis is usually supportive and aimed at relieving the symptoms and/or complications; it includes:
- Nothing by mouth (NPO)
- Analgesics
- Gastric decompression

- Hydration
- Antibiotics (after appropriate cultures are done)
- Anticholinergics (decrease pancreatic activity, both metabolic and secretory; also reduce gastric acid secretion)
- Short-acting insulin (treat hyperglycemia and reduce stress on the pancreas)
- Antacids (neutralize gastric acid)
- Vigorous resuscitation efforts (if the clinical picture is severe)
- Surgery if a pancreatic abscess or biliary obstruction is suspected.

6. Nursing considerations

a. Vital Signs. Monitor and record vital signs frequently, including temperature and blood pressure. Report sudden changes and/or trends.

b. Volume expansion. Administer and closely monitor fluid replacement. If blood products are required, follow hospital protocols for transfusions.

c. Gastric decompression. Assure patency and proper functioning of the gastric tube (see Chapter 9) in an effort to prevent gastric acids and air from entering the intestines. If antacid therapy is begun, follow protocol for clamping the gastric tube.

d. NPO. The patient should be kept NPO until pain-free. Clear liquids then may be resumed and the diet advanced as tolerated.

e. Respiratory status. Closely monitor breath sounds, respiratory rate, chest roentgenograms, and arterial blood gases for indications of pulmonary involvement (atelectasis, effusions, etc.).

f. Positioning. Frequent turning (every 2 hours) and positioning the patient in semi-Fowler's position will promote lung expansion and decrease enzyme and fluid accumulation in the lungs.

g. Analgesia. Meperidine hydrochloride (Demerol) may be an effective analgesic. Avoid using morphine, as it increases the resting tone of Oddi's sphincter; this can cause more pain and may elevate the patient's amylase and lipase levels.

h. Laboratory studies. Assure that laboratory studies are performed as ordered. Monitor trends in enzymes, calcium, electrolytes, CBC, amylase, and lipase levels. Follow and report serum glucose levels, as treatment with insulin may be required.

i. Teaching the patient. Considerable instruction may be required, prior to the patient's discharge, concerning alcohol intake and dietary habits.

B. Paralytic ileus

Paralytic, or adynamic, ileus is an intestinal obstruction (resulting from decreased or ineffective peristalsis) that causes gas and/or fluid to accumulate in the affected portion of the bowel. It differs from mechanical bowel obstruction in that the former involves no physical or mechanical obstruction.

1. Etiology

Paralytic ileus may be caused by metabolic, humoral, and neural factors. It is precipitated or aggravated by numerous clinical problems (Table 7-3).

TABLE 7-3

FACTORS THAT PRECIPITATE OR AGGRAVATE PARALYTIC ILEUS

Shock	Myocardial infarction
Sepsis	Anesthesia
Bowel ischemia/infarct	Pneumonia
Retroperitoneal hematoma	Premature feeding
Respiratory failure	Pancreatitis
Hypoxia	Peritonitis
Acid-base imbalance	Spinal cord injury
Electrolyte imbalance	Premature removal of
Pelvic or vertebral fractures	gastric tube

2. Assessment

Since paralytic ileus is such a common complication, it is important to identify patients at risk. Be on the lookout for the classic heralding sign — abdominal distention. If the ileus is severe or goes undiagnosed, the patient may appear septic, with fever, elevated WBC, and/or shock. Also assess for:

- Bowel sounds (diminished or absent)
- Vomiting/increased gastric drainage (gastric rather than feculent material)
- Hiccups (indications of increased pressure on the patient's diaphragm)
- Pain (usually dull, diffuse, and continuous but possibly more severe than the pain of surgery).

3. Diagnosis

Radiographic studies usually reveal gas and/or fluid distending the stomach, small bowel, and colon.

4. Treatment

If paralytic ileus can't be prevented (the best treatment), the following measures are taken:

- Gastric/intestinal/rectal decompression
- Correction of electrolyte and acid-base imbalances
- Hydration via intravenous therapy
- NPO
- Ambulation (when possible).

5. Nursing considerations

a. Prevention. Avoid premature feeding or premature removal of gastric tube before return of normal bowel sounds, flat abdomen, and passage of flatus.

b. Decompression. Be sure that gastric, intestinal, or rectal tubes are patent and functioning properly (see Chapter 9 for description).

c. Bowel sounds. Monitor bowel sounds frequently. Notify physician of significant changes, particularly the development of a "silent" abdomen in a patient who previously had bowel sounds.

d. Abdominal girth. Measure and record abdominal girth every 4 to 6 hours.

e. Intake/output. Closely monitor and record fluid intake and all output (gastric, bowel, urinary). If gastric drainage is excessive, it may be necessary to replace an equal amount of fluid to maintain hydration. Also monitor and record gastric pH. Antacid treatment may be required if the pH is 5 or less.

f. Laboratory studies. Make sure that all lab studies are performed as ordered. Closely monitor acid-base and electrolyte studies.

QUIZ

1. Describe the difference between mechanical bowel obstruction and paralytic ileus: _____
   _____.

2. The two most common causes of acute pancreatitis are _____ and _____.

3. The classic sign of paralytic ileus is _____.

4. Bowel sounds with paralytic ileus may be
   _____
   or _____.

5. _____ is the best treatment for paralytic ileus.

6. _____ is the most important aspect of treatment for paralytic ileus.

7. _____ is the most common symptom of pancreatitis.

8. The pain of pancreatitis is often relieved by

_____ and/or _____ .

9. _____ and/or _____
levels are usually elevated with acute pancreatitis.

ANSWERS

1. With a paralytic ileus there is no mechanical obstruction of the bowel; there is a paralysis of peristalsis.

2. Alcoholism; biliary tract disease.

3. Distention.

4. Diminished; absent.

5. Prevention.

6. Decompression.

7. Pain.

8. Any of the following: fasting, knee-chest position, vomiting, leaning forward.

9. Amylase, lipase, glucose, WBC, sedimentation rate.

CHAPTER

8

Surgical Problems

OBJECTIVES

After completing this chapter, you will be able to:

1. *Name the two most common symptoms of surgical abdominal problems*

2. *State at least one cause of each of the surgical abdominal problems*

3. *Describe the type of pain, or pain pattern, associated with each specific problem.*

A. Appendicitis

Appendicitis, defined as inflammation of the vermiform appendix, is one of the most common surgical problems in the abdomen. Acute appendicitis occurs most frequently between the ages of 2 and 40.

1. Etiology

The precise etiology of appendicitis is still under question. It is generally thought, however, that the appendix becomes obstructed — for example, by calculi or adhesions. This obstruction leads to decreased venous return, edema, and hemorrhage, resulting in a bacterial invasion of the appendix.

After the appendix becomes inflamed, it can become gangrenous and may rupture if not promptly removed. Perforation is seen most commonly before the age of 10 and after the age of 40; it can create symptoms of local or general peritonitis. Chronic appendicitis may cause a low-grade inflammatory process.

2. Assessment

The symptomatology of appendicitis may be atypical, especially in an elderly patient, who might have other intra-abdominal diseases, or in a very young patient, who might be incapable of recognizing and describing his symptoms accurately. Assess the patient for the following:

a. Pain. Abdominal tenderness is the most consistent finding in all ages. The classic symptoms of appendicitis begin with severe periumbilical or epigastric pain that localizes in the right lower quadrant (McBurney's point) after 6 to 12 hours. The pain may be described as colicky or crampy and may increase in intensity. However, the pain pattern may not be specifically identifiable as due to appendicitis. There may be generalized or rebound tenderness. If rupture occurs, look for abdominal rigidity resulting from spasms of the rectus muscle and a palpable right lower quadrant mass, indicative of an abscess.

b. Nausea/vomiting. Anorexia follows the onset of pain and frequently leads to nausea and vomiting.

c. Fever. Usually the patient has a low-grade fever (below 101°F or 38°C). If perforation occurs, a more significant elevation will be seen.

d. Laboratory studies. The patient with appendicitis *usually* (but not always) has a white blood cell count greater than 10,000.

e. Ascites. Ascites may develop as a result of chronic appendicitis with resulting intra-abdominal inflammation.

3. Preoperative nursing considerations

During the preoperative period, the patient is limited to bed rest and permitted to take nothing by mouth. Nursing responsibilities during this time include the frequent monitoring and recording of vital signs (blood pressure, pulse, respiration, temperature); the administration of analgesia; the provision of psychological support; and, if required, a simple explanation of the surgical procedure to be performed. If clinical signs suggest that the patient has suffered a rupture, gastric suction is warranted. Finally, make sure that a consent to surgery has been obtained.

4. Diagnosis/treatment

The diagnosis of appendicitis is usually suggested by the presence of pain, vomiting, and fever. In the absence of these classic signs, the diagnosis may be more difficult. If there is serious cause for doubt, the patient may be hospitalized and observed for several hours. However, since the treatment for appendicitis is early removal of the appendix, it is much safer to perform a laparotomy and find a normal appendix than to delay surgery and risk the complications that arise from a ruptured one.

5. Postoperative nursing considerations

Routine postoperative care of the appendectomy patient includes the administration of analgesics as needed and care of the wound. Watch for signs of inflammation, since wound infection may occur—especially if the appendix ruptured before it could be removed. Antibiotic therapy is usually instituted only in patients with appendiceal rupture or abscess. In any case, the dressings must be changed regularly and sterile technique observed. Where recovery is uneventful, the patient is usually allowed early ambulation. Sutures are generally removed 5 to 7 days postoperatively.

B. Mechanical bowel obstruction

Mechanical bowel obstruction (MBO) can be defined as physical blockage of the intestinal lumen. This blockage can occur as a result of an extrinsic, intrinsic, or intraluminal factor. The obstruction may be complete or incomplete, transient or persistent, and strangulating or nonstrangulating. MBO may occur in the small or large intestine; however, the latter is less common.

1. Etiology

Frequent causes and/or precipitating factors of MBO are listed in Table 8-1. Obstruction of the small bowel is most commonly caused by adhesions; that of the large bowel is most often due to carcinoma.

2. Assessment

a. Pain. A patient with MBO experiences episodes of sharp, colicky, or cramping pain in the mid- to lower abdomen. The pain-free intervals become shorter as the obstruction progresses.

TABLE 8-1

CAUSES AND PRECIPITATING FACTORS OF
MECHANICAL BOWEL OBSTRUCTION

Adhesions	Abscess
Hernia	Endometriosis
Gallstones	Inflammatory bowel disease
Tumor	Ischemia
Fecal or barium impaction	Hematoma
Diverticulitis	Foreign body
Carcinoma	

b. Distention. Abdominal distention occurs in both small and large bowel obstructions and usually causes diffuse abdominal tenderness.

c. Bowel sounds. Bowel sounds are usually hyperactive; however, there may also be occasional periods when no sounds are audible.

d. Nausea/vomiting. Nausea and vomiting, which may be mild to moderate, occur as intestinal contents back up into the stomach. The vomitus is therefore feculent.

e. Bowel movements. If the obstruction is complete, the patient may be constipated or have no bowel movements. Diarrhea and the passage of flatus usually indicate a partial obstruction.

f. Possible gangrene. If the MBO results in circulatory impairment of the bowel or if it goes untreated, the involved bowel may become gangrenous. Observe this patient for the following signs:
- Severe, continuous, localized pain
- Abdominal distention with marked tenderness
- Persistent vomiting (stools/vomitus may be bloody or melenic, or they may contain occult blood)
- Diminished or absent bowel sounds
- Tachycardia
- Fever
- Dehydration
- Elevated WBC
- Sepsis; peritonitis
- Shock.

3. Diagnosis

The clinical assessment and patient's history will usually suggest the diagnosis of MBO. Additional diagnostic tools include roentgenogram of the abdomen, proctoscopy, and barium studies. The WBC may be normal or elevated with a shift to the left. Electrolyte and BUN studies are needed to evaluate the degree of dehydration.

4. Treatment

Treatment includes the following measures:
- Proximal decompression
- IV volume expansion
- Correction of electrolyte imbalances
- Antibiotics
- Surgery, if indicated to remove the obstruction.

5. Nursing considerations

Closely assess and monitor this patient for signs of complications such as peritonitis (see section E, below), sepsis, and shock. Nursing responsibilities also include:

a. Vital signs. Closely monitor and record vital signs (blood pressure, pulse, respiration, temperature), since this patient may become hemodynamically unstable.

b. Hydration. Assist with and monitor the effects of IV therapy and volume expansion. Closely monitor fluid intake and output.

c. Decompression. Assure patency and proper functioning of gastric and/or intestinal tubes to promote decompression of the bowel proximal to the blockage. Aspiration of bowel or gastric contents into the lungs can be a lethal complication.

d. Laboratory studies. Assure that all lab studies are performed as ordered. Follow BUN and electrolytes (to evaluate effects of hydration) and the WBC (for potential sepsis).

e. Antibiotics. Administer antibiotics as ordered.

f. Vomitus/stool. Test all vomitus and/or stool for occult blood.

C. Hernias

A hernia is defined as a musculofascial disruption or defect that allows abdominal fat, a section of the peritoneum, and/or a loop of bowel to protrude visibly. The incidence of hernias is significantly higher in males than in females.

1. Etiology

A hernia may result from one of three causes:
- A congenital failure of a normal opening to close
- An acquired weakness secondary to old age, injury, debilitating illness, or prolonged abdominal distention (pregnancy, tumors, obesity, ascites)
- Increased intra-abdominal pressure, as from coughing, straining, or heavy lifting.

2. Assessment

a. Symptoms. The patient is usually the first to notice the hernia and may describe it as a lump that pops out when he strains or coughs. The patient may or may not experience accompanying pain at the site.

b. Location. Hernias occur in several locations; they may, for example, be inguinal, femoral, umbilical, or incisional.

c. Type. During your physical examination, it will be necessary to determine whether the hernia is reducible or nonreducible. A reducible hernia is one that will disappear when gentle pressure is applied to the hernial sac. A strangulated or incarcerated hernia is one that will not reduce with gentle pressure.

3. Diagnosis

The diagnosis of a hernia, its type, and its location is made from the physical examination and the patient's history.

4. Treatment

The treatment of choice is surgical repair of the muscle and fascia (either by suturing or by insertion of a synthetic graft) before the hernia reaches the stage of strangulation. If, however, the hernia is already incarcerated, the portion of necrotic or ischemic bowel must be resected and the hernial defect repaired. If surgery on a reducible hernia is not immediately possible, a truss may be worn temporarily to prevent recurrence.

5. Nursing considerations

Postoperative care of the herniorrhaphy patient includes monitoring vital signs, administration of analgesics as needed, and wound care. Application of an ice bag to the incision may help relieve discomfort.

Urinary retention may be a problem, especially after the repair of an inguinal hernia. Therefore, carefully monitor fluid intake and output and watch for symptoms of urinary tract involvement.

Patients usually are allowed to ambulate within 24 to 36 hours after surgery. Before discharge, they should be warned to avoid physical stress and told that heavy exertion is prohibited for approximately 10 weeks. Return to ordinary activities and routines should be careful and gradual.

D. Acute cholecystitis

Gallstones are a significant health problem affecting approximately 10 percent of the male and 20 percent of the female population. Women over age 40 usually have the highest incidence of this disease.

1. Etiology

Acute cholecystitis is a complication that occurs when the cystic duct becomes obstructed by gallstones. The gallbladder becomes enlarged with bile and inflamed tissue. An attack of acute cholecystitis may progress to local perforation with formation of an abscess, or to generalized peritonitis. There may also be a series of repeated attacks. The attacks may last as long as 7 to 10 days, but most patients experience spontaneous remission of symptoms within 48 to 72 hours.

2. Assessment

Slow onset with intermittent episodes of right upper quadrant pain is characteristic of acute cholecystitis. The gallbladder is frequently palpable and there may be hepatic enlargement.

a. Mild inflammation. The patient with mild inflammation usually describes indigestion, nausea/vomiting, colicky right upper quadrant pain, and tenderness radiating to the back or base of the right scapula. There may be voluntary guarding.

b. Severe inflammation. With a more severe attack, the colicky pain is more intense and may be aggravated by movement. (This patient lies motionless.) Fever, muscle spasms, local rebound tenderness, and Murphy's sign may be present as well. Perforation of the gallbladder should be suspected if the abdominal tenderness and pain become generalized.

3. Diagnosis

a. Laboratory studies. Most patients have elevated SGOT and SGPT levels, which peak and then fall to normal or near normal within 3 to 5 days. The WBC is usually elevated to 12,000 to 15,000; elevated bilirubin, lipase, alkaline phosphatase, and amylase are common. The urinary amylase may be elevated as well.

b. Other studies. The diagnosis of gallstones is best accomplished by the use of ultrasound, but gallstones may be visualized on an abdominal roentgenogram in approximately 15 percent of patients. Intravenous cholangiography is the recommended diagnostic tool when acute cholecystitis is suspected. This study will outline a normal gallbladder and fail to visualize it during an acute attack.

4. Treatment

a. Hospitalization. Hospitalization is recommended to assure careful, frequent monitoring.

b. Antibiotics. Antibiotic therapy is controversial and usually reserved for a patient with a secondary bacterial infection, one whose attack persists beyond 5 days, or one whose condition deteriorates.

c. Infusions. Correction of fluid and electrolyte imbalances secondary to poor oral intake and vomiting may be necessary.

d. NPO. The patient is kept NPO; gastric suction may be needed for prolonged nausea or vomiting.

e. Analgesia. Analgesia can usually be provided by pentazocine (Talwin). The use of morphine or meperidine (Demerol) is to be avoided, as they may increase ductal pressure.

f. Surgery. Early surgery to avoid the complications of perforation is recommended.

5. Complications

The most common complication of acute cholecystitis is perforation of the gallbladder. The three forms of perforation are local rupture with abscess formation, generalized perforation with peritonitis, and rupture into a hollow viscus with fistula formation. All three forms of perforation require surgical intervention.

6. Nursing considerations

- Closely monitor and record vital signs, including temperature
- Accurately record volume replacement and output (urinary, bowel, gastric)
- Administer analgesics and antibiotics as prescribed
- Maintain patency and functioning of the gastric tube (see Chapter 9) to facilitate removal of gastric contents and prevent mucosal damage
- Make sure that laboratory studies are performed as ordered; monitor results for sudden changes or trends
- Provide the necessary physical and psychological support before diagnostic studies or surgery.

E. Peritonitis

Peritonitis—inflammation of the peritoneum, the membranous lining of the abdominal cavity—may be classified as primary, spontaneous, or secondary.

1. Etiology

a. General causes. The five general causes of peritonitis are:

- Rupture or perforation of a viscus or associated structure
- Female genital tract infection

- Puncture of the abdominal wall
- Infection of blood or lymphatic systems
- Surgical contamination.

b. Primary peritonitis. Primary peritonitis is due to an acute or subacute invasion by bacteria such as *Escherichia coli*, streptococci, pneumococci, or gonococci. It may stem from infections in the kidneys, uterus, bladder, ovaries, and/or GI tract.

c. Secondary peritonitis. Secondary peritonitis results from irritation by blood, bile, stool, urine or enzymes. Causes of secondary peritonitis include ruptured appendix, trauma, cirrhosis, ruptured peptic ulcer, ectopic pregnancy, chole-cystitis, and diverticulitis.

2. Assessment

The clinical picture of peritonitis varies in severity, depending on the location of the source and on whether the inflammation is localized or generalized. In general, assess the patient for:

a. Pain. The pain experienced may be generalized or diffuse and increasing in severity, or it may be localized to a specific region. This pain is usually constant and may be aggravated by coughing or moving. There can be rebound tenderness. The patient may obtain some relief by lying motionless in the supine position, with knees drawn up.

b. Bowel sounds. Paralytic ileus, with diminished or absent bowel sounds, commonly accompanies peritonitis. Percussion elicits tympanic sounds, which arise from the gas trapped in the intestine.

c. Nausea/vomiting. Anorexia is common; nausea/vomiting frequently is the first sign of peritonitis.

d. Fever. The patient is usually febrile, with an elevated WBC and tachycardia.

e. Ascites. Ascites may develop as a result of the inflammatory process.

3. Diagnosis

The clinical picture and patient history should be sufficient evidence to diagnose secondary versus primary peritonitis and even possibly the causative factor. Peritoneal aspiration, laparoscopy, culturing, and urinalysis may be helpful in determining the causative factor. The priority with secondary peritonitis, however, is deciding whether or not the patient requires emergency abdominal surgery. Determining the specific cause of the peritonitis is important; however, valuable time may be lost and the patient's life put at increased risk if surgery is significantly delayed. This would occur if, for example, a ruptured appendix were causing the peritonitis. Frequently, it will be impossible to determine the cause of the peritonitis without a laparoscopy or laparotomy.

4. Treatment

Treatment of secondary peritonitis is often surgery first and diagnosis of the cause second. Postoperatively, the patient usually requires IV therapy, gastric decompression, antibiotics, and any specific therapy directed toward the causative factor. Treatment of primary peritonitis is usually supportive and includes an antibiotic regimen.

5. Nursing considerations

a. Hemodynamics. Closely monitor and record vital signs, temperature, and urinary output.

b. Hydration. Assist with and monitor the effects of volume expansion.

c. Decompression. Keep the patient NPO. Assure proper functioning and patency of the gastric tube to promote decompression and prevent aspiration.

d. Antibiotics. Administer antibiotics as ordered.

e. Complications. Monitor and assess the patient for potential complications such as abscess formation, evisceration, and respiratory involvement.

f. Postoperative care. Depending on the causative factor, there may be additional nursing responsibilities postoperatively: monitoring and caring for abdominal drains, surgical wounds, and so on.

QUIZ

1. List, in correct sequence, the three major symptoms of appendicitis: _____, _____, and _____.

2. True or false: Appendicitis rarely occurs after the age of 10.

3. True or false: An appendectomy is indicated only when the appendix has ruptured.

4. True or false: If untreated, a mechanical bowel obstruction may result in shock, gangrene, and sepsis.

5. The pain caused by a mechanical bowel obstruction is usually _____ and occurs _____.

6. A hernia is classified as _____ or _____.

7. _____ is the most common complication of acute cholecystitis.

8. A urinary tract infection, cirrhosis, and an ectopic pregnancy are all potential causes of _____.

9. Match the most appropriate symptoms with the surgical problem on the left.

Appendicitis _____
MBO _____
Peritonitis _____
Cholecystitis _____

a. Nausea/vomiting, diffuse abdominal tenderness, ileus

b. Epigastric pain that localizes at McBurney's point

c. Hyperactive bowel sounds, feculent vomitus

d. Colicky pain aggravated by movement

10. The two most common symptoms of a surgical abdominal problem are _____ and _____.

ANSWERS

1. Pain, nausea/vomiting, fever.
2. False. Appendicitis occurs most frequently between the ages of 2 and 40.
3. False. The treatment of choice for appendicitis is early removal of the appendix, before it ruptures.
4. True.
5. Colicky or crampy; in episodes.
6. Reducible; nonreducible (strangulated, incarcerated).
7. Rupture of the gallbladder.
8. Peritonitis.
9. Appendicitis _b_
   MBO _c_
   Peritonitis _a_
   Cholecystitis _d_
10. Pain; nausea/vomiting.

9

Tubes/Drains

OBJECTIVES

After completing this chapter, you will be able to:

1. State the purpose of each tube and drain

2. State one potential complication of each tube and drain

3. List three nursing actions for maintenance of each tube and drain.

A. Salem sump

Table 9-1 summarizes the Salem sump's features.

1. Nature and purpose

The Salem sump is a gastric tube used primarily to irrigate and remove accumulated secretions from the stomach, for decompression, and to administer nutritional fluids and medications.

2. Mechanics

The tubing itself is made of radiopaque clear plastic and is disposable, being intended for one-time-only use. Its double lumen comprises a suction port (large) and air vent (small), designed for use with continuous suction (30 to 40 mm Hg) or intermittent gastric suction (80 to 120 mm Hg).

3. Additional equipment

In using the Salem sump, you'll need the following additional equipment:
- Gloves and lubricant
- Emesis basis
- Glass of water and straw
- Irrigation syringe
- Stethoscope
- Tape.

4. Procedure

a. Preparation

1. Explain procedure briefly, but honestly, to enlist patient's cooperation.

2. Place patient in Fowler's position when possible.

3. Take distal end of tube and measure from tip of patient's nose to his ear lobe, then down to the sternal tip. (This approximates the necessary length of tubing.)

4. Lubricate entire tube to facilitate passage.

b. Insertion. Inserting a Salem tube is a nursing action unless the patient has esophageal surgery/trauma, gastric surgery/trauma, rhinorrhea, facial nasal fractures, or a basal skull fracture.

TABLE 9-1

SALEM SUMP

Purpose
Decompression
Administration of nutritional support/medication
Irrigation

Mechanics
Radiopaque
Clear plastic
Double lumen (large, suction port; small, air vent)
Air vent system
Disposable
Continuous or intermittent gastric suction

Additional equipment
Gloves and lubricant
Emesis basin
Glass of water and straw
Irrigation syringe
Stethoscope
Tape

1. Gently insert tube into nostril. When it reaches the posterior pharynx, instruct patient to swallow small sips of water to facilitate passage into the esophagus.

2. Continue slow insertion of tube to premeasured distance.

3. When tube is in place, gently aspirate gastric contents from large lumen. Instill a small amount of air while auscultating below the ribs, left of the midline, to ensure proper placement.

4. Remove entire tube if patient becomes cyanotic or is in obvious respiratory distress.

5. Secure tube to patient's nose with nonallergenic tape to prevent dislodgement.

c. Maintenance

1. Irrigate large lumen with 30 ml of normal saline and small lumen with 30 ml of air at least every 2 hours (while suction is applied) to maintain tube patency and prevent mucosal damage. If gastric contents back up into the air-vent lumen, the tube may be coiled or blocked or the proxi-

mal end may be below the level of the heart. Elevate the proximal end and irrigate both the suction lumen and the air vent. If these measures fail, remove entire tube and reinsert.

2. Check tube placement every 8 hours (with shift assessment) and prior to every feeding or administration of medication.

3. Monitor nares for signs of irritation. (Tube may be placed in opposite nostril or in mouth if irritation occurs.)

4. Assess and record amount and character of gastric drainage. Include output in I/O totals.

5. Look for, report, and document any obvious or occult blood in gastric contents.

6. Assess, report, and document gastric pH. It should be at least 5.0.

7. Ensure that gastric tube drains at least 50 ml/shift. If output is less, tube may not be functioning properly.

8. Never clamp or occlude air-vent lumen while suction is applied. A blocked lumen creates a vacuum that may cause gastric mucosal damage.

9. When transporting patient without suction, *never* plug the large lumen; this may lead to aspiration if he vomits. Attach a large irrigation syringe with the plunger retracted to allow for escape of gastric contents.

d. Removal

1. Remove tube slowly. Expect patient to gag or retch during removal.

2. Discard tube.

5. Potential complications

These include irritation or ulceration of the gastric mucosa, irritation of the nares, and sinusitis.

B. Levin tube

The salient features of Levin tubes are briefly summarized in Table 9-2.

1. Nature and purpose

The Levin tube is designed primarily for administration of medication and nutritional fluids. Extreme caution must be

TABLE 9-2

LEVIN TUBE

Purpose
Administration of medication/nutritional support
Decompression (requires extreme caution)

Mechanics
Radiopaque
Clear plastic
Single lumen
No air-vent system
Disposable
Low-pressure suction (30-40 mm Hg) if used for decompression

Additional equipment
Gloves and lubricant
Emesis basin
Glass of water and straw
Irrigation syringe
Stethoscope
Tape

exercised if the Levin tube is used for decompression, as there is no air-vent system.

2. Mechanics

The tubing is made of radiopaque clear plastic and is disposable (like the Salem sump, it's intended for one-time-only use). It has a single lumen with no air-vent system and must be used with low-pressure suction (30 to 40 mm Hg) when used for decompression.

3. Additional equipment

Use of the Levin tube requires the following additional equipment:
- Gloves and lubricant
- Emesis basin
- Glass of water and straw
- Irrigation syringe
- Stethoscope
- Tape.

4. Procedure

a. Preparation. Preparation is the same as for the Salem sump.

b. Insertion. Inserting a Levin tube is a nursing action unless the patient has esophageal surgery/trauma, gastric surgery/trauma, rhinorrhea, facial/nasal fractures, or a basal skull fracture.

The procedure is the same as for the Salem sump, except that aspiration may be difficult without an air-vent system.

c. Maintenance. Again, follow the same procedures as for the Salem sump. In addition:

1. Exercise extreme caution if this tube is used for suction/decompression, as there is no air-vent system to break the vacuum. Gastric mucosal irritation or ulceration is a likely complication. Vigilant monitoring of tube patency is essential.

2. Between feedings and medication doses, or during transport, attach the tube to straight drainage to allow for escape of gastric contents should the patient vomit; this will help prevent aspiration.

d. Removal. As with the Salem sump, remove the Levin tube slowly, and then discard it. Expect the patient to gag or retch during removal.

5. Potential complications

These include irritation/ulceration of the gastric mucosa, irritation of the nares, and sinusitis.

C. Cantor tube

See Table 9-3 for points to remember concerning the Cantor tube.

1. Nature and purpose

The Cantor tube, used for intestinal intubation (decompression), is weighted at the distal end so that it will not stop in the stomach, but pass through it into the duodenum.

TABLE 9-3

CANTOR TUBE

Purpose
Intestinal decompression

Mechanics
Radiopaque
Silicone rubber
Single lumen (suction holes proximal to bag)
Mercury balloon at distal end
Low-pressure suction

Additional equipment
Gloves and lubricant
21-gauge needle
10-ml syringe
Mercury
Cotton-tipped applicator
McGill forceps

2. Mechanics

The single-lumen tubing is made of radiopaque silicone rubber. It is weighted with a mercury balloon and has suction holes proximal to the balloon.[*]

3. Additional equipment

You'll need the following equipment to assist in placing a Cantor tube:
- Gloves and lubricant
- 21-gauge needle
- 10-ml syringe
- Mercury
- Cotton-tipped applicator
- McGill forceps.

4. Procedure

a. Preparation

1. Explain procedure briefly, but honestly, to enlist patient's cooperation.

[*] *Proximal* and *distal* in this chapter refer to the perspective of the nurse or other caregiver, not that of the patient.

2. Place patient in Fowler's position when possible.

PHYSICIAN follows instructions for instilling mercury into balloon.

3. Lubricate tube to facilitate passage.

b. Insertion. This is the physician's responsibility. You are to assist the physician as needed.

PHYSICIAN inserts tube to marked letter "s," indicating placement in stomach. Tube is inserted gradually (2 to 4 inches at a time) while the patient is turned and positioned; peristalsis facilitates passage into the duodenum.

1. Do not tape tube to patient's face. Loosely coil remaining tubing and attach to patient's gown.

PHYSICIAN confirms proper placement by roentgenogram.

c. Maintenance

1. Irrigate tube frequently to assure patency. Aspiration may be difficult because of the tube's placement in the intestine.

2. Monitor nares for signs of irritation.

3. Assess and record amount and character of intestinal drainage. Include output in I/O totals.

4. Allow mercury to pass normally if balloon ruptures; ingested mercury is not absorbed and therefore is not toxic.

d. Removal. This is the physician's responsibility. Assist as needed.

1. If tube is nondisposable type, remove and return mercury-filled bag to the pharmacy for disposal; return tube to sterile supply for sterilization.

5. Potential complications

These include irritation of the nares; also, intestinal necrosis/rupture may result from distention of mercury bag with intestinal gas/air.

D. Miller-Abbott tube

Table 9-4 lists the attributes of the Miller-Abbott tube.

1. Nature and purpose

The double-lumen Miller-Abbott intestinal tube has an inflatable latex balloon at its distal end. It is used to treat obstructions of the small intestine, as an aid to diagnosis, to provide intestinal decompression, and to administer medications and nutritional fluids.

2. Mechanics

One lumen is intended for use with suction or for administration of medication or nutrition into the intestine. The other channel is solely for instillation of mercury into the balloon. This red rubber tube is radiopaque and reusable; it may be autoclaved.

3. Additional equipment

When using the Miller-Abbott tube, you'll need the following additional equipment:
- Gloves and lubricant
- 10-ml syringe
- Mercury
- Cotton-tipped applicator
- McGill forceps.

TABLE 9-4

MILLER-ABBOTT TUBE

Purpose
Treatment of obstruction
Diagnosis
Intestinal decompression
Administration of medications/nutritional support

Mechanics
Double lumen (balloon port; suction/feeding port)
May be autoclaved
Radiopaque
Red rubber with latex balloon

Additional equipment
Gloves and lubricant
10-ml syringe
Mercury
Cotton-tipped applicator
McGill forceps

4. Procedure

a. Preparation
- Explain procedure briefly, but honestly, to enlist patient's cooperation.
- Clearly label both balloon and suction ports.
- Place patient in Fowler's position when possible.
- Lubricate balloon and tube to facilitate passage.

b. Insertion. Insertion is the physician's responsibility. Assist as needed.

PHYSICIAN inserts tube. Once tube is in place in stomach, physician instills 3 to 10 ml of mercury into balloon port. Tube is inserted gradually (2 to 4 inches at a time) while the patient is turned and positioned; peristalsis facilitates passage into the duodenum.

1. Do not tape tube to patient's face. Loosely coil remaining tubing and attach to patient's gown.

PHYSICIAN confirms proper placement by roentgenogram.

c. Maintenance
1. Monitor nares for signs of irritation.
2. Use extreme caution when administering medications and feedings. If tube feeding liquid is inadvertently inserted into the balloon port, the distended balloon may cause intestinal necrosis or rupture.
3. If balloon ruptures, mercury will not be absorbed and therefore will not be toxic; allow it to pass normally.
4. Frequent irrigation of suction port will help assure patency of tube. Aspiration may be difficult because of the tube's placement in the intestine.

d. Removal. It's the physician's responsibility to remove a Miller-Abbott tube. Assist as needed.

PHYSICIAN aspirates all mercury from balloon port.
1. Send mercury to pharmacy for disposal.
2. Return tube to sterile supply for sterilization

5. Potential complications

These include irritation of the nares as well as intestinal necrosis or rupture.

TABLE 9-5

SENGSTAKEN-BLAKEMORE TUBE

Purpose
Gastric and/or esophageal tamponade
Differentiation between gastric and esophageal bleeding sites

Mechanics
Triple lumen (gastric balloon, esophageal balloon, gastric aspiration port)
Radiopaque
May be autoclaved

Additional equipment
Gloves and lubricant
Tracheal suction apparatus
Irrigation syringe
Traction device (Blakemore football helmet)
Foam rubber padding
Clamps with rubber protectors

E. Sengstaken-Blakemore tube

Table 9-5 outlines the main features of this device.

1. Nature and purpose

This three-channel tube with two inflatable balloons is designed for gastric and esophageal tamponade and for use in differentiating between gastric and esophageal bleeding sites. It also provides for gastric suction, to aspirate the contents of the stomach.

2. Mechanics

The first balloon is inflated in the stomach to hold the tube in place and exert pressure on the cardiac sphincter. The second, long balloon goes into the esophagus to press against bleeding varices. The third tube leads from the stomach to a suction apparatus. The tubing is radiopaque. Both it and the balloons are reusable and may be autoclaved.

3. Additional equipment

Use of a Sengstaken-Blakemore tube usually requires the following:
- Gloves and lubricant
- Tracheal suction apparatus

- McGill forceps
- Irrigation syringe
- Traction device (Blakemore football helmet)
- Foam rubber padding
- Clamps with rubber protectors.

4. Procedure

a. Preparation

1. Explain procedure briefly, but honestly, to enlist patient's cooperation.

2. Place patient in Fowler's position when possible.

3. Ensure that all tubes are clearly marked.

4. Before insertion, submerge both balloons under water to check for leaks.

5. Lubricate tube and balloons to facilitate passage.

6. Have tracheal suction turned on at bedside.

b. Insertion. The physician inserts a Sengstaken-Blakemore tube. Assist physician as needed.

PHYSICIAN inserts entire tube, either nasally or orally, until gastric balloon is in stomach, and inflates gastric balloon with 25 to 50 ml of air.

1. Aspirate through gastric port.

When position of tube is confirmed by roentgenogram, PHYSICIAN further inflates balloon with 200 to 250 ml of air and clamps securely.

PHYSICIAN applies traction so tube rests firmly against the cardioesophageal junction. Use of football helmet, face mask, or other such device will maintain traction.

2. Apply foam padding around tube at nares level to prevent pressure on nares. Tape tube to chin guard.

PHYSICIAN inflates esophageal balloon with 25 to 45 mm of mercury as measured by manometer. Lowest amount of necessary pressure is used to tamponade bleeding.

3. Clamp esophageal balloon securely.

c. Maintenance

1. Make sure both esophageal and gastric balloons remain inflated and are securely clamped.

2. Measure esophageal balloon pressure by manometer every 15 to 30 minutes. Deflate esophageal balloon after 24

to 48 hours of continuous use; deflate gastric tube after 48 hours of use to prevent mucosal necrosis.

3. Patient cannot swallow oral secretions. Frequent suctioning of mouth and nose and frequent mouth care will therefore be necessary.

4. Closely monitor respiratory status. Keep scissors at bedside at all times. If gastric balloon ruptures, traction will pull tube upward and occlude patient's airway. Should this occur, immediately cut all tubes and remove entire device.

5. A gastric suction tube may be placed above the level of the esophageal balloon to remove secretions and drainage and prevent aspiration.

d. Removal. This is the physician's responsibility.

PHYSICIAN releases traction, removes air from both balloons, and then removes tube. Assist as needed.

1. Return tube to sterile supply for sterilization.

5. Potential complications

These include esophageal rupture due to pressure/necrosis, aspiration pneumonia, airway obstruction/respiratory distress, and nasal irritation.

F. Mercury-weighted feeding tubes

Table 9-6 summarizes the pertinent features of these tubes.

TABLE 9-6
MERCURY-WEIGHTED FEEDING TUBES

Purpose
Administration of nutritional fluids into duodenum or jejunum via infusion pump

Mechanics
Soft, flexible rubber
Mercury tip at distal end
Feeding tube with distal mercury tip
Radiopaque
Guide wires for insertion on some brands
May be disposable or reusable (autoclavable)

Additional equipment
Gloves and lubricant
Glass of water and straw
Infusion pump
Tape

1. Nature and purpose

Flexible, weighted feeding tubes are used to administer nutritional fluids into the duodenum or jejunum. Delivery is regulated by an infusion pump.

2. Mechanics

Made of soft, flexible rubber and fitted with a mercury tip at the distal end, these tubes may be either disposable or reusable (autoclavable). The tubes have holes at the distal end, and some brands have guide wires to aid insertion.

3. Additional equipment

When using a feeding tube, you'll need the following:
- Gloves and lubricant
- Glass of water and straw
- Infusion pump
- Tape.

4. Procedure

a. Preparation

1. Explain procedure briefly, but honestly, to enlist patient's cooperation.
2. Place patient in Fowler's position when possible.
3. Lubricate tube to facilitate passage.

b. Insertion. Feeding tubes are inserted by the physician. Assist as needed.

1. Instruct patient to swallow when mercury weight is at posterior pharynx.

PHYSICIAN inserts initial two-thirds of tube. Remainder of tube is gradually inserted over several hours; as patient is positioned and turned, peristalsis facilitates passage of remaining third of tube into proximal jejunum or distal duodenum. PHYSICIAN confirms position of tube by roentgenogram before feedings can be started.

2. When desired position is obtained, securely tape tube to patient's face.

c. Maintenance

1. If feeding is stopped, irrigate tube with 20 ml of water. Plug tube with attached cap. Before resuming feedings, irrigate again as above.

2. Use a 50-ml syringe to irrigate tube. A smaller syringe places excessive pressure on the tube, which may cause it to balloon out and rupture.

d. Removal

1. Gently remove tube and return mercury bolus to pharmacy.

2. Discard tube if disposable; if not, return to sterile supply.

5. Potential complications

These include sinusitis/nasal necrosis (rare) and passage of tube into tracheobronchial tree.

G. Needle-catheter jejunostomy

Table 9-7 outlines this device's features.

1. Nature and purpose

The needle-catheter jejunostomy provides a route for administration of nutritional fluids directly into the jejunum. Delivery is regulated by an infusion pump.

TABLE 9-7

NEEDLE-CATHETER JEJUNOSTOMY

Purpose
Immediate postoperative jejunal feeding via infusion pump

Mechanics
Kit or separately packaged 24-inch intracatheter and 14-gauge needle
Radiopaque
Disposable

Additional equipment
Gastric decompression tube and suction apparatus (may be used simultaneously)
Infusion pump
Dressings

---

2. Mechanics

This device comprises 2 feet of radiopaque, disposable intracatheter tubing and a 14-gauge needle, supplied either separately or as a kit.

3. Additional equipment

Feeding via a needle-catheter jejunostomy requires the following additional equipment:
* Gastric decompression tube with suction apparatus (may be used simultaneously)
* Infusion pump
* Dressings.

4. Procedure

a. Preparation and insertion. These are the physician's responsibilities. The catheter is inserted during surgery directly into the lumen of the jejunum and pursestring-sutured to the intestinal wall. The catheter is then tunneled out through the abdominal wall and sutured to the skin. A secure dressing is applied.

b. Maintenance. PHYSICIAN performs first dressing change after 72 hours.

   1. Change dressing every 48 to 72 hours, using aseptic technique.

   2. Monitor patient for signs of peritonitis or subcutaneous tissue inflammation or infection at jejunostomy site.

   3. Administer formula diet via infusion pump as ordered.

c. Removal. This tube is removed by the physician; assist as needed.

   1. Discard catheter.

5. Potential complications

These include skin inflammation at jejunostomy site, subcutaneous abscess formation, and generalized peritonitis. (If catheter becomes dislodged, feedings are infused into the peritoneal cavity.)

TABLE 9-8

PENROSE DRAIN

Purpose
Drainage by gravity

Mechanics
Soft rubber tubing, various widths

Additional equipment
Sterile safety pin
Dressings

H. Penrose drain

Table 9-8 describes the pertinent attributes of Penrose drains.

1. Nature and purpose

The Penrose drain is designed to facilitate drainage from abdominal surgical wounds by means of gravity flow.

2. Mechanics

The drain is a soft, flat rubber tube available in various widths. Drainage material usually is absorbed by a gauze dressing.

3. Additional equipment

Use of the Penrose drain requires the following:
  • Sterile safety pin
  • Dressings.

4. Procedure

a. Preparation and insertion. These are the physician's responsibilities. The drain is inserted during surgery near the operative site, through a separate stab incision.

PHYSICIAN may place a sterile safety pin horizontally across the drain at skin level to prevent it from sliding back into the abdomen.

b. Maintenance

1. Assure sterile management of drain and dressing.

2. Monitor skin integrity at insertion site. Record/report assessment findings.

3. Assess and record amount and character of drainage through or around drain. Include amount of drainage in I/O records.

4. If drainage is excessive, apply sterile colostomy bag over the drain and secure. This helps to control and monitor the amount of drainage accurately; it also prevents potential skin irritation.

c. Removal. PHYSICIAN usually advances the drain outward by about 1 inch each day to promote outward granulation and prevent formation of tract infection.

5. Potential complications

These include infection and retrograde sliding of the drain.

I. Hemovac and similar drains

Table 9-9 summarizes the pertinent features of these devices. (The Hemovac is the prototype, and best known, of this kind of drain; others have appeared on the market more recently.)

1. Nature and purpose

These closed-wound suction devices are designed to remove thin fluids from surgical sites by means of gentle suction.

2. Mechanics

The drain consists of a small plastic spring-loaded drum attached to a long plastic tube with drainage holes in its distal end. As the spring gradually uncoils, it creates nega-

TABLE 9-9

HEMOVAC AND SIMILAR DRAINS

Purpose
Drainage of thin fluid from surgical site

Mechanics
Spring-loaded drainage drum
Long drainage catheter with distal drainage holes
Creates negative pressure in cavity

Additional equipment
Dressings

---

tive pressure inside the drum, which draws fluid through the tubing.

3. Additional equipment

Dressings are required.

4. Procedure

a. Preparation and insertion. These are the physician's responsibilities. The drain is inserted through a stab incision adjacent to the surgical site during surgery, and sutured in place.

b. Maintenance

1. Assure sterile management of drain and dressing.

2. Monitor skin integrity at insertion site. Record/report assessment findings.

3. Maintain negative pressure and prevent clotting by collapsing drum periodically.

4. Empty drum at least every 8 hours and record/report amount and character of drainage. Include amount of drainage in I/O records.

5. Monitor patency of drainage catheter. Record and report any clots; these may clog the drain and possibly give rise to infection.

c. Removal. The drain is removed by the physician, usually 48 to 72 hours after surgery, when drainage has declined substantially, or when the drain becomes clotted. The device is removed all at once.

5. Potential complications

Infection is the principal complication.

J. Shirley sump

Table 9-10 summarizes the particular features of the Shirley sump.

1. Nature and purpose

The Shirley sump, used in conjunction with continuous suction, provides drainage of fluid and pus from abdominal surgical sites.

TABLE 9-10

SHIRLEY SUMP

Purpose
Drainage of fluid, pus

Mechanics
Tube with distal drainage holes
Drainage port and air-vent system
Air-vent port: yellow cap with four vent holes
Creates equalized negative pressure (air-vent system
    prevents organ damage from suction vacuum)

Additional equipment
Dressings
Suction system
Irrigation syringe

2. Mechanics

This disposable device consists of a tube with drainage holes at the distal end, a drainage port, an air-vent system, and an air-vent port (cap with four vent holes) at the proximal end. Its air-vent system creates equalized negative pressure, preventing organ damage from the suction vacuum.

3. Additional equipment

Use of the Shirley sump requires the following:
  • Dressings
  • Suction apparatus
  • Irrigation syringe.

4. Procedure

a. Preparation and insertion. PHYSICIAN inserts the Shirley sump during surgery near the operative site through a separate, adjacent stab incision. It is then sutured into place.

b. Maintenance
  1. Keep air-vent holes and cap uncovered and dry to assure proper functioning of vent system.
  2. Help assure patency and proper functioning of sump by aspirating it periodically with an irrigation syringe.

PHYSICIAN may irrigate if necessary to remove a blockage in the drain; this is not a nursing action.

3. Assure sterile management of sump/dressing.

4. Change entire suction apparatus every 24 hours to prevent retrograde contamination.

5. Monitor skin integrity around insertion site. Record/report assessment findings.

6. Assess and record amount and character of drainage. Include drainage amount in I/O records.

c. Removal. PHYSICIAN removes Shirley sump when drainage has decreased significantly or has stopped.

5. Potential complications

Infection is the principal complication.

K. Saratoga sump

See table 9-11 for a list of points concerning this device.

1. Nature and purpose

The Saratoga sump provides for the drainage of blood, pus, and viscous fluids in large amounts from abdominal surgical sites. It is intended to form a wide tract to promote drainage.

TABLE 9-11

SARATOGA SUMP

Purpose
Drainage of large quantities of blood, pus, viscous fluid
Formation of wide tract to promote drainage

Mechanics
Argyl drain
Two channels (inner, drainage; outer, air vent)
Continuous suction required
Creates equalized negative pressure (air-vent system
   prevents organ damage from suction vacuum)

Additional equipment
Suction apparatus
Irrigation syringe
Dressings

2. Mechanics

The Saratoga sump is a disposable drain with two channels, an inner one for drainage and an outer one for venting. Continuous suction is required. The equalized negative pressure created by the sump's air-vent system prevents organ damage due to the suction vacuum.

3. Additional equipment

When using the Saratoga sump, you'll need the following additional equipment:
- Suction apparatus
- Irrigation syringe
- Dressings.

4. Procedure

a. Preparation and insertion. PHYSICIAN inserts the Saratoga sump during surgery near the operative site through a separate, adjacent stab incision. The drain is then sutured into place.

b. Maintenance

1. Assure that proximal air-vent holes are patent and uncovered.

2. Help assure patency and proper functioning of drainage channel by aspirating it periodically with an irrigation syringe.

PHYSICIAN may irrigate if necessary to remove a blockage in the drain; this is not a nursing action.

3. Assure sterile management of drain/dressing.

4. Change entire suction apparatus every 24 hours to prevent retrograde contamination.

5. Monitor skin integrity around insertion site. Report/record assessment findings.

6. Assess/record amount and character of drainage. Include amount in I/O record.

c. Removal. PHYSICIAN removes Saratoga sump when drainage has decreased significantly or has stopped. PHYSICIAN may cut tube and use it as a passive drain, which may gradually be advanced outward over several days.

TABLE 9-12

DAVAL SUMP

Purpose
Drainage of large quantities of blood, pus, viscous fluid
Irrigation of body cavity through irrigation port

Mechanics
Disposable silicone drain
Three ports (drainage, air vent, irrigation)
Requires continuous suction
Creates equalized negative pressure (air-vent system prevents
  organ damage from suction vacuum)

Additional equipment
Suction apparatus
Irrigation syringe
Dressings

5. Potential complications

Infection is the principal complication.

L. Daval sump

See Table 9-12 for the pertinent features of this device.

1. Nature and purpose

The Daval sump provides for the drainage of blood, pus, and
viscous fluids in large amounts from abdominal surgical
sites. It also can be used for irrigating a body cavity through
its irrigation port.

2. Mechanics

The Daval sump is a disposable silicone drain with three
ports, for drainage, venting, and irrigation. It requires continuous suction. Like the Shirley and Saratoga sumps, it creates equalized negative pressure; its air-vent system prevents
organ damage from the suction vacuum.

3. Additional equipment

Use of the Daval sump requires the following additional
equipment:
  • Suction apparatus

- Irrigation syringe
- Dressings.

4. Procedure

a. Preparation and insertion. PHYSICIAN inserts the Daval sump during surgery near the operative site through a separate stab incision. It is then sutured into place.

b. Maintenance

1. Be sure cap on air-vent port remains dry and patent. Remove and replace if it becomes damp or wet.

2. Help assure patency and proper functioning of drainage channel by aspirating it periodically with an irrigation syringe.

PHYSICIAN may irrigate if necessary to remove a blockage in the drain; this is not a nursing action.

3. Be sure irrigation port is capped shut when not in use.

4. Assure sterile management of drain and dressing.

5. Change entire suction apparatus every 24 hours to prevent retrograde contamination.

6. Monitor skin integrity around insertion site. Record/report assessment findings.

7. Assess and record amount and character of drainage. Include amounts in I/O record.

c. Removal. PHYSICIAN removes Daval sump when drainage has decreased significantly or has stopped.

5. Potential complications

Infection is the principal complication.

QUIZ

1. Two complications that may result from the Salem sump are:_____ and _____.

2. True or false: Reflux of gastric material into the Salem air-vent port may indicate that the proximal end of the sump is too high.

3. True or false: Intestinal rupture is a potential complication of using the Miller-Abbott tube.

4. True or false: Ingestion of mercury, resulting from rupture of the Cantor balloon, is a medical emergency.

5. The Penrose drain utilizes _____ to promote drainage.

6. The Saratoga is a _____ -channel drain.

7. The three lumens of the Sengstaken-Blakemore tube are designed for _____, _____, and _____.

8. True or false: Irrigation of an abdominal drain is a nursing responsibility.

9. _____ is the most serious, life-threatening complication of using the Sengstaken-Blakemore tube.

10. Two complications of a needle-catheter jejunostomy are: _____ and _____.

ANSWERS

1. Any of the following: sinusitis, nasal irritation, gastric mucosal irritation/ulceration.

2. False. The proximal sump end must be elevated to prevent gastric reflux through the air vent.

3. True.

4. False. Mercury is not absorbed and therefore is not toxic.

5. Gravity.

6. Double.

7. An esophageal balloon, a gastric balloon, gastric suction.

8. False. Irrigation is the physician's responsibility.

9. Airway obstruction.

10. Any of the following: subcutaneous abscess formation, insertion site infection, peritonitis.

CHAPTER

10

Selected Medications

OBJECTIVES

After completing this chapter, you will be able to:

1. *List two actions of vasopressin (Pitressin), cimetidine (Tagamet), and antacids*

2. *List six potential side effects of vasopressin*

3. *Describe two nursing implications for each drug discussed.*

A. Vasopressin

1. Actions and indications

a. Actions. Vasopressin injection (Pitressin) is an antidiuretic hormone that concentrates urine by increasing water reabsorption in the renal tubules. It also stimulates contraction of smooth muscle in the GI tract and vascular bed (venules, small arterioles, and capillaries).

b. Indications. Vasopressin may be ordered for control of severe GI bleeding, to help decrease shadows before abdominal radiography, for prevention or treatment of postoperative abdominal distention, and for control of diabetes insipidus.

2. Potential side effects

Possible side effects — rare with low doses — include urticaria, anaphylaxis, diaphoresis, nausea/vomiting, bronchial constriction, increased peristalsis, increased sphincter pressure, decreased gastric secretions, myocardial infarction, cardiac arrhythmias, bradycardia, decreased cardiac output, increased pulmonary arterial pressure, and hypertension.

3. Nursing implications
- Patient should be on cardiac monitor
- Monitor electrolytes, urine output, mental status, and vital signs
- Give IV via central line; administration through peripheral line may cause skin vasoconstriction leading to necrosis
- Dosage should be tapered off to prevent rebleeding
- Doses above 0.4 unit/minute may increase morbidity and mortality and do not increase effectiveness.

4. Dose

For control of GI bleeding in adults, initial dose is 0.2 unit/minute and should produce optimal reduction in blood flow in 20 to 30 minutes.

B. Cimetidine

1. Actions and indications

a. Actions. Cimetidine (Tagamet) is a histamine H_2 receptor antagonist that inhibits basal gastric acid secretion as well as gastric acid secretion stimulated by food, caffeine, histamine, or insulin.

b. Indications. This drug is indicated for short-term therapy of active duodenal ulcers and for prevention of their recurrence.

2. Potential side effects

Cimetidine may cause reversible increases in plasma creatinine levels. Rare side effects include dizziness, rash, somnolence, and mild, transient diarrhea.

3. Nursing implications

- Give IV push injections slowly, over 1 to 2 minutes; rapid bolus may cause hypotension or cardiac arrhythmias
- Give IV infusions over 15 to 20 minutes
- Do not give oral cimetidine simultaneously with any antacid, as antacid may interfere with absorption of cimetidine; concomitant administration (with cimetidine and antacid doses staggered) is acceptable, however.

4. Dose

Usual dose is 300 mg every 6 hours; not to exceed 2,400 mg every 24 hours.

C. Antacids

1. Actions and indications

a. Actions. Common antacids include sodium bicarbonate, calcium carbonate (Titralac), magnesium hydroxide (Mylanta II, Maalox), aluminum hydroxide gels (Amphojel), magaldrate (magnesium aluminum hydrate; Riopan), and various combinations of these ingredients available over the counter under numerous trade names. They coat the gastric mucosa and have a nonsystemic buffering action that neutralizes or reduces gastric acid, thus reducing the pain associated with excessive gastric acid.

b. Indications. Antacids are used in peptic ulcer disease, hiatal hernias, and gastric hypersecretory disorders.

2. Potential side effects

Antacids may cause constipation, nausea/vomiting, diarrhea, phosphate deficiency (aluminum hydroxide), or hypermagnesemia (magaldrate).

3. Nursing implications
- Watch for constipation and diarrhea
- Consider sodium content when giving to patients with renal impairment, hypertension, or dietary sodium restriction
- Effectiveness varies with stomach emptying time, but generally lasts 30 to 60 minutes
- Advisable to avoid giving simultaneously with other oral drugs, as antacid may inhibit other drugs' absorption
- If administering antacid down gastric tube, follow procedure for clamping, irrigating, etc.
- If giving antacid as chewable tablet, make sure patient chews tablet completely before swallowing.

4. Dose

The dose of antacids is individualized, depending on the pathology and degree of pain.

QUIZ

1. Myocardial infarction, urticaria, and hypertension are potential side effects of _____.

2. Optimal blood flow reduction usually occurs _____ after the administration of vasopressin.

3. The usual dose of cimetidine is _____ every _____ hours, not to exceed _____ per 24 hours.

4. Three potential side effects of antacids are: _____ , _____ , and _____.

5. Antacids may be given in conjunction with _____ to help relieve _____.

6. Vasopressin administered in doses greater than 0.4 units/minute may increase _____.

ANSWERS

1. Vasopressin.
2. 20 to 30 minutes.
3. 300 mg, 6; 2,400 mg.
4. Any of the following: constipation, nausea, vomiting, diarrhea, phosphate deficiency, hypermagnesemia.
5. Cimetidine; pain.
6. Morbidity, mortality rates.

CHAPTER

11

Procedures

OBJECTIVES

After completing this chapter, you will be able to:

1. Describe the purpose of each procedure discussed

2. List two nursing actions for the "preparation," "procedure," and "follow-up" phases of each procedure

3. List two complications of each procedure.

A. Introduction

The following diagnostic procedures are the responsibilities of the physician; however, the nurse must act as the patient's advocate and assist the physician during each step of these procedures.

B. Peritoneal lavage

1. Purpose

This procedure is used to determine the possible presence of intra-abdominal injury and the need for laparotomy. Peritoneal lavage does not identify the specific organ injured and is not performed if the patient has a penetrating abdominal injury.

2. Equipment

- Peritoneal lavage tray
- Dialysis catheter and trocar
- 1-liter bottle of normal saline solution (NSS) and intravenous tubing
- Suture material (per physician request)
- Two red-top blood sample tubes
- Foley catheter tray
- Gastric decompression tube and irrigation syringe
- Razor.

3. Procedure

a. Preparation

1. Briefly, but honestly, explain procedure to enlist patient's cooperation.

2. Place patient in supine position.

3. Insert urinary catheter and gastric decompression tube to prevent potential complications.

4. Assure that abdomen is cleanly shaved.

5. Flush NSS through IV tubing and hang at bedside.

6. Assure that all medical personnel involved observe sterile procedure policy (mask, gloves, hat).

b. During procedure

1. Assist physician as needed.

PHYSICIAN drapes patient and performs abdominal surgical scrub. He then injects local anesthetic containing epinephrine. PHYSICIAN incises lateral to umbilicus down to peritoneum, then punctures peritoneum with trocar-enforced catheter. Hemostasis must be maintained to avoid false-positive lavage results.

A left lower quadrant incision may be necessary if there are previous abdominal scars, if the patient is pregnant, or if the abdomen is significantly distended. (The left lower quadrant site is preferred to avoid future confusion with an appendectomy scar.)

PHYSICIAN removes trocar and advances catheter downward toward pelvis. He gently aspirates from catheter. If gross blood is obtained, no fluid is infused and patient undergoes laparotomy.

2. If no blood is aspirated, connect IV tubing to catheter and rapidly infuse NSS. (Solution should be warmed before use if patient is hypothermic.)

3. During infusion, place patient in slight Trendelenburg position (if neurologically safe) to bathe diaphragm. Inform patient that it is normal to experience feelings of pressure or fullness during infusion.

4. When infusion is complete, invert bottle and place on the floor. Disconnect IV tubing and reinsert into air-vent port. (This breaks the vacuum and promotes lavage return by gravity.)

5. While lavage fluid is returning, patient may be placed in slight reverse Trendelenburg position to facilitate drainage from the abdominal cavity.

6. Withdraw and send sample of return fluid for red and white cell counts. (Amylase and bilirubin analysis may be performed if physician requests.)

c. **Follow-up.** Upon receipt of cell count results, PHYSICIAN removes catheter. Positive results (frank blood; red cell count $\geq$100,000; white cell count $\geq$500; amylase $\geq$200; presence of bile, fecal matter, bacteria) dictate need for laparotomy;

wound is temporarily packed. If results are negative, wound is sutured and dressed.

1. Document procedure and effects on patient.

4. Potential complications

These include puncture of (distended) bladder, intestines, or mesenteric vessels as well as peritoneal infection.

C. Endoscopy

1. Purpose

This procedure is used for direct visualization and/or suction of the esophageal, gastric, and duodenal mucosa as well as to obtain specimens (by brushing).

2. Additional equipment

- Sedative and/or muscle relaxant (as ordered)
- ECG monitor at bedside
- Suction apparatus at bedside
- Emergency "crash" cart at bedside.

3. Procedure

a. Preparation

1. Identify patients who are at risk for complications (elderly or unstable patients as well as those with pre-existing coagulopathy or pulmonary disease).

2. Patient should have nothing by mouth at least 6 hours before procedure to eliminate food particles from esophagus and prevent aspiration.

3. Briefly, but honestly, explain procedure to enlist patient's cooperation and decrease anxiety.

4. Make sure patient's consent is obtained in writing (per hospital policy).

5. Remove patient's dentures.

6. Position patient as ordered (supine with neck hyper-extended, left lateral recumbent, or Fowler's).

b. During procedure

1. Provide reassurance and explanations.

PHYSICIAN may use anesthetic spray to decrease gag reflex

and discomfort; 5 to 15 minutes should be allowed for optimal effect.

2. Assure patient that sensation of swollen tongue and throat is normal, as is inability to swallow; have tracheal suction at bedside to remove saliva.

3. Administer sedative and/or muscle relaxant as ordered by physician.

4. Make sure emergency equipment is nearby for treatment of potential complications.

5. Report and document changes or trends in patient's status to physician performing procedure.

6. Be aware that cramping pain is normally experienced as scope passes through pylorus.

c. Follow-up

1. Keep patient NPO until gag reflex returns (approximately 3 to 4 hours).

2. Administer analgesics as ordered to minimize any throat discomfort.

3. Document procedure and effects on patient.

4. Monitor patient for at least 24 hours for potential complications; document and report any complaints of chest or gastric pain.

4. Potential complications

- Esophageal perforation (see Chapter 6)
- Aspiration pneumonia
- Cardiovascular problems: ventricular tachycardia, atrial fibrillation, myocardial infarction, hypotension, cardiac arrest
- Medication reactions
- Aggravation of bleeding
- Respiratory problems: hypoxia, respiratory distress, respiratory arrest.

D. Colonoscopy

1. Purpose

This procedure is performed in order to visualize the large intestine directly, to obtain biopsy specimens, and to excise polyps from the colon.

2. Additional equipment
- Fluoroscope
- Sedative and/or muscle relaxant (as ordered).

3. Procedure

a. Preparation

1. Patient should receive only liquids for 24 to 48 hours prior to procedure, as ordered.

2. Administer cathartics as ordered.

3. Administer cleansing enemas as ordered.

4. Report and document effects of cathartics and/or cleansing enemas.

5. Briefly, but honestly, explain procedure to enlist patient's cooperation and decrease anxiety.

6. Be sure that consent is obtained (per hospital policy).

7. Position patient on left side for beginning of procedure.

b. During procedure. Colonoscopy is an embarrassing procedure for the patient. Provide a professional atmosphere and assurance to the patient to help preserve his dignity.

1. Provide reassurance and explanations.

2. Administer sedatives and/or muscle relaxants as ordered by physician.

3. Assist with draping of patient.

4. Reposition patient as physician requests during performance of procedure.

5. Report and document patient's expressed feelings or complaints about procedure.

6. Assure patient that feelings of abdominal cramping are normal when air is inserted through the scope.

c. Follow-up

1. Clean patient and equipment as appropriate.

2. Document procedure and effects on patient.

3. Monitor patient for rectal bleeding and abdominal pain; record and report these symptoms.

4. Potential complications

These include rupture of the bowel and hemorrhage.

E. Sigmoidoscopy

1. Purpose

This procedure is performed in order to visualize the sigmoid colon and rectal lumen directly, to obtain biopsy specimens, and to remove polyps.

2. Additional equipment

- Sedative and/or muscle relaxant (as ordered)
- Suction apparatus.

3. Procedure

a. Preparation

1. Restrict patient's diet for 24 hours prior to procedure if so ordered by physician.

2. Administer enemas 1 hour prior to procedure as ordered by physician.

3. Briefly, but honestly, explain procedure to enlist patient's cooperation and decrease anxiety.

4. Be sure that consent is obtained (per hospital policy).

5. Position patient as requested by physician (Sims's knee-chest).

b. During procedure.
This is an embarrassing procedure for the patient. Provide a professional atmosphere and assurance to the patient to help preserve his dignity.

1. Assist with draping of patient.

2. Provide reassurance and explanations; assure patient that feeling the urge to defecate is normal and instruct patient to take slow, deep breaths through the mouth as scope is inserted.

3. Administer sedation and/or muscle relaxants as ordered by physician.

4. Report and record patient's expressed feelings or complaints about procedure.

5. Have suction apparatus at bedside for use with sigmoidoscope.

c. Follow-up

1. Clean patient and equipment as appropriate.
2. Document procedure and effects on patient.

3. Assess for, report, and record any rectal bleeding or abdominal pain.

4. Potential complications

These include rupture of the bowel and hemorrhage.

F. Upper gastrointestinal series (with small bowel exam)

1. Purpose

This procedure is used to visualize the esophagus, stomach, and small intestine, using barium sulfate as the contrast medium.

2. Additional equipment

- Barium and cup.

3. Procedure

a. Preparation

1. Keep patient NPO after midnight prior to procedure.
2. Do not give purgatives prior to procedure.
3. Briefly, but honestly, explain procedure to enlist patient's cooperation and decrease anxiety.

b. During procedure

1. Provide reassurance and explanations.
PHYSICIAN instructs patient when to drink barium, how much, and when to stop drinking.
2. Position patient as ordered.

c. Follow-up

1. Administer cathartics as ordered.
2. Monitor stools to ensure constipation does not result from barium retention.
3. Inform patient that stools will be white for 24 to 72 hours if no cathartics are given.

4. Potential complications

These include adverse reaction to the contrast medium and constipation.

G. Barium enema

1. Purpose

This procedure is used to visualize the colon, cecum, and appendix, using a barium sulfate solution as the contrast medium.

2. Additional equipment
- Bedpan or bathroom nearby
- Towels.

3. Procedure

a. Preparation

1. Make sure the large bowel is clear, for best results.

2. Provide liquid diet and administer cathartics as ordered the day prior to procedure.

3. Administer cleansing enemas the night before and the morning of the procedure.

4. Keep patient NPO for the procedure.

5. Briefly, but honestly, explain procedure to enlist patient's cooperation and decrease anxiety. (It will be necessary for the patient to retain the barium enema to achieve the best results.)

6. Position patient as ordered (lateral recumbent).

b. During procedure. A barium enema can be an embarrassing procedure as the patient may not be able to retain the barium as requested; provide a professional atmosphere and assurance to the patient to help preserve his dignity.

1. Provide reassurance and explanations; assure patient that the feelings of pressure/fullness, cramping, and urge to defecate are normal.

2. Position patient as requested during procedure.

c. Follow-up

1. Assist patient to bathroom or onto bedpan to expel the barium solution.

2. Administer cleansing enemas or cathartics as ordered and encourage high fluid intake to expedite expulsion of barium and rehydration.

3. Monitor and record stools to ensure that constipation or impaction does not result from retained barium.

4. Inform patient that stools will be white for 24 to 72 hours after the procedure if no cathartics are given.

4. Potential complications

These include reaction to the contrast medium and constipation or impaction.

QUIZ

1. True or false: Peritoneal lavage diagnoses specific intra-abdominal organ injury.

2. True or false: Penetrating abdominal injuries do not require peritoneal lavage.

3. True or false: Peritoneal lavage should never be performed on a pregnant woman.

4. Match the appropriate complication on the right with the diagnostic procedure on the left.

   a. Endoscopy _____
   b. Sigmoidoscopy _____
   c. Peritoneal lavage _____
   d. Barium enema _____
   e. Upper GI series _____

   1. Reaction to contrast medium
   2. Hemorrhage
   3. Cardiac arrest
   4. Ruptured bladder
   5. Fecal impaction

ANSWERS

1. False. Peritoneal lavage determines only the presence or absence of intra-abdominal injury.

2. True.

3. False. Peritoneal lavage can be performed in the left lower quadrant in a pregnant patient.

4. a. 3. b. 2. c. 4. d. 5. e. 1.

12

Selected Laboratory Studies

OBJECTIVES

After completing this chapter, you will be able to:

1. Identify the enzymes found chiefly in the liver

2. State normal values for the laboratory tests discussed

3. State the difference between direct and indirect bilirubin levels.

A. Serum glutamic-oxaloacetic transaminase

This enzyme, commonly abbreviated SGOT, is also known as aspartate aminotransferase (AST).

1. Normal physiology

SGOT is an intracellular enzyme located predominantly in the heart and liver. Smaller amounts are found in the kidneys, red blood cells, skeletal muscle, and pancreatic tissue.

2. Pathology

Intracellular SGOT is released into the blood after cellular injury or death. The serum level is in direct proportion to the number of injured cells and the time interval between injury and testing.

3. Laboratory values

a. Normal. Normal values range from 5 to 20 units/ml.*

b. Time course. SGOT levels become elevated 8 hours after injury, reach a peak 24 to 36 hours after injury, and return to normal in 4 to 6 days.

c. Abnormal. Values of 1,000 units/ml or more represent severe liver necrosis or severe fulminating hepatitis. Values between 40 and 100 units/ml are typical of cirrhosis.

B. Serum glutamic-pyruvic transaminase

This enzyme, commonly abbreviated SGPT, is also known as alanine aminotransferase (ALT).

1. Normal physiology

SGPT is an intracellular enzyme found in highest concentrations in the liver.

2. Pathology

Cellular injury or death causes SGPT to be released into the blood.

---

*The normal values given in this chapter are measured according to the standards of the laboratory at the University of Maryland Hospital. Enzyme activities expressed in units are equivalent to micro-international units.

3. Laboratory values

Normal values range from 5 to 36 units/ml.

C. Alkaline phosphatase

1. Normal physiology

Alkaline phosphatase, sometimes abbreviated ALP or alk. phos., is found in bone, the liver, intestines, and placenta.

2. Pathology

Cellular injury causes alkaline phosphatase to be released into the blood.

3. Laboratory values

a. Normal. Normal values range from 15 to 70 units/ml.

b. Abnormal. Alkaline phosphatase levels more than five times normal represent obstructive jaundice. Since alkaline phosphatase is not elevated in hepatocellular jaundice, its measurement is a useful means of distinguishing hepatocellular from obstructive jaundice.

D. Lactate dehydrogenase

1. Normal physiology

This enzyme, abbreviated LDH, is found in greatest concentrations in the heart, kidneys, liver, skeletal muscle, and red blood cells. Isoenzymes of LDH can be separated to determine the organ or tissue of their origin.

2. Pathology

Serum levels of LDH reflect damage to the tissues or organs already mentioned.

3. Laboratory values

a. Normal. Normal values range from 30 to 120 units/ml.

b. Abnormal. Slight elevations indicate chronic viral hepatitis or hepatic malignancy.

c. Spurious. Hemolyzed blood samples will give falsely elevated LDH results.

E. Bilirubin

1. Normal physiology

Bilirubin is a by-product of normal hemoglobin breakdown. A small portion is used in bile formation; the rest must be excreted. Most bilirubin (the plasma-bound or unconjugated form) is excreted in the feces; only about 1 percent (the soluble or conjugated form) is excreted in the urine.

2. Pathology

Elevated serum bilirubin levels reflect one of three disorders:
- Excessive production of bilirubin in relation to the liver's ability to excrete it
- Obstruction of excretion by the liver
- A problem with excretion itself.

3. Laboratory values

a. Total. Total serum bilirubin normally does not exceed 0.1 to 1.2 mg/dl.

b. Direct. The direct bilirubin test measures soluble (conjugated) bilirubin, excreted in the urine, which normally does not exceed 0.3 mg/dl. This test is specific for obstructive jaundice and hepatobiliary disease (mild liver disease).

c. Indirect. The indirect bilirubin test measures plasma-bound (unconjugated) bilirubin, which is not excreted in the urine. Normal values range from 0.1 to 1.0 mg/dl. This test is an important indicator of jaundice in general; more specific tests must be done to identify the type and cause of jaundice.

F. Prothrombin time

1. Normal physiology

Prothrombin is a glycoprotein, found in plasma, that is converted to thromboplastin during the clotting process. Conversion to thromboplastin relies on hepatic synthesis of other clotting factors and intestinal absorption of vitamin K.

2. Pathology

Death or injury of the liver cells that synthesize clotting factors V, VII, and X, vitamin K deficiency, or administration of anticoagulants slows or prevents the conversion of pro-thrombin to thromboplastin.

3. Laboratory values

Normal prothrombin time (PT) is 12 to 14 seconds. Prolonged prothrombin time indicates the extent of disease or damage, but not its nature or cause. Proper evaluation of PT results requires control values.

QUIZ

1. _____ is found primarily in the liver.

2. The enzymes are released into the circulatory system after _____.

3. Match the lab test on the left with the normal value on the right.

    a. LHD _____   **1.** 15 to 70

    b. SGOT _____   **2.** 5 to 36

    c. Alk. Phos. _____   **3.** 12 to 14 seconds

    d. SGPT _____   **4.** 5 to 20

    e. Direct bilirubin _____   **5.** 30 to 120

    f. Indirect bilirubin _____   **6.** Up to 0.3

    g. PT _____   **7.** 0.1 to 1.0

ANSWERS

1. SGPT.

2. Cellular injury or death.

3. a. 5.   b. 4.   c. 1.   d. 2.   e. 6.   f. 7.   g. 3.

GLOSSARY

Ascites — excessive accumulation of fluid in the peritoneal cavity resulting from altered venous return, obstruction of lymphatic drainage, or electrolyte imbalance

Autodigestion — digestion of tissues by the organ's own secretions

Coffee-ground emesis — emesis that resembles coffee grounds in color and texture; occurs when blood is present in vomitus; usually indicates bleeding has slowed or stopped

Cullen's sign — ecchymosis around the umbilicus, resulting from dissection of retroperitoneal blood into the abdominal wall

Feculent — containing or having the odor of feces

Greater omentum — double fold of peritoneum suspended from the greater curvature of the stomach downward to cover the intestines

Grey Turner's sign — ecchymosis over the flank area, which results from dissection of retroperitoneal blood into the abdominal wall

Hematemesis — vomitus containing blood and often clots

Hematochezia — fresh red blood in the feces

Icterus — jaundice

Kehr's sign — pain (from irritated diaphragm) referred to the left shoulder tip

Lesser omentum — fold of peritoneum that extends from the lesser curvature of the stomach to the transverse fissure of the liver

Ligament of Treitz — suspensory ligament attached to the junction of the jejunum and duodenum

McBurney's point — in appendicitis, area of tenderness on the line between the umbilicus and 1 to 2 inches above the right anterior superior iliac spine

Melena — black, tarry stool or vomitus resulting from the mixture of intestinal juices and blood

Mesentery — peritoneal folds that connect the intestines with the posterior abdominal wall

Murphy's sign — pain produced upon inspiration while gentle palpation is performed in the right subcostal area

Rebound tenderness — pain or tenderness experienced when the gentle pressure of palpation is released

Referred pain — pain experienced in a region some distance from its point of origin (example: Kehr's sign)

Rugae — folds of mucous membranes in the interior stomach

Spider nevi — branches of dilated capillaries on the skin that resemble a spider

Villi — small, finger-like projections in the small bowel

ADDITIONAL TEST QUESTIONS

1. Match the function in the left column to the correct organ in the right column:

    a. Secretion of bile _____   **1.** Liver

    b. Absorption of water _____   **2.** Large bowel

    c. Production of heparin _____   **3.** Gallbladder

    d. Blood storage _____   **4.** Spleen

2. The patient should be in the _____ position for abdominal examination.

3. List at least five things to look for when assessing the abdominal skin:

4. _____ is performed before _____ to avoid disturbing bowel sounds.

5. Bowel sounds heard 20 to 30 times/minute are considered _____.

6. True or false: The absence of bowel sounds indicates an intra-abdominal injury in the trauma patient.

7. When evaluating gastric drainage, assess _____, _____, _____, _____, and _____.

8. During the act of vomiting, the patient's heart rate usually _____.

9. Two complications of excessive nausea/vomiting/diarrhea are _____ and _____.

10. Anesthesia, pancreatitis, and the use of meperidine hydrochloride (Demerol) may all precipitate _____.

11. Two complications of peptic ulcer disease are
_____ and _____.

12. The primary goal of treatment for the patient with a UGI bleeding episode is _____.

13. Arteriography is not a useful diagnostic tool for esophageal varices because _____
_____.

14. _____ is the preferred diagnostic tool for UGI bleeding.

15. Alcoholism and biliary tract disease are the most common causes of _____.

16. Four laboratory studies that should be performed when pancreatitis is suspected are _____, _____, _____, and _____.

17. One nursing responsibility for the patient with a gastric decompression tube is _____, which may be accomplished by frequent _____.

18. The use of morphine should be avoided in the patient with pancreatitis because it may increase _____ and _____ levels.

19. Absent bowel sounds, diffuse abdominal pain, distention, and vomiting are common symptoms of
_____.

20. One of the most common abdominal surgical emergencies is _____.

21. _____ is the most common symptom of appendicitis and is usually experienced at
_____.

22. An MBO most commonly occurs in the _____ intestine as a result of _____.

23. _____ bowel sounds are characteristic of MBO.

24. An incarcerated hernia is one that _____.

25. _____ is a potential complication after _____ hernial repair.

26. A patient with cholecystitis usually lies _____.

27. The initial priority with peritonitis is _____
_____.

28. Match the functions on the left with the tube or drain on the right.

    a. Tamponade _____   **1.** Hemovac

    b. Decompression _____   **2.** Saratoga

    c. Irrigation _____   **3.** Blakemore-Sengstaken

    d. Administration   **4.** Cantor
       of feedings _____   **5.** Salem

    e. Drainage of thin   **6.** Needle-catheter
       fluid _____   jejunostomy

    f. Drainage of blood,
       pus _____

29. Match the potential complication on the right with the tube/drain on the left.

    a. Blakemore-Sengstaken _____   **1.** Infection

    b. Daval _____   **2.** Airway obstruction

    c. Salem sump _____   **3.** Intestinal rupture

    d. Miller-Abbott _____   **4.** Aspiration

    e. Levin _____   **5.** Sinusitis

30. Mercury poisoning is a potential hazard with:

    a. Cantor _____

    b. Shirley _____

    c. Miller-Abbott _____

    d. None of the above _____

31. Frequent mouth care and suctioning are necessary when a Sengstaken-Blakemore tube is in place because
_____.

32. The normal SGPT value is _____.

33. The normal total bilirubin level is _____.

34. True or false: Peritoneal lavage should never be performed on an unconscious trauma patient.

35. A _____ and a _____ should be inserted prior to peritoneal lavage.

36. Myocardial infarction, respiratory distress, aspiration pneumonia, and esophageal perforation are potential complications of _____.

37. During a colonoscopy, the patient may experience _____ when air is inserted through the scope.

38. Two complications of a sigmoidoscopy are _____ and _____.

39. Two complications of a barium enema are _____ and _____.

40. Name two functions of the spleen:

41. Cimetidine may be used prophylactically in patients at risk for _____.

42. Intravenous vasopressin (Pitressin) may be used for a patient with esophageal varices because it _____
_____.

43. Antacids may be administered concomitantly with cimetidine to _____.

44. Optimal gastric pH should be maintained at _____.

45. List six potential complications after abdominal trauma:

ANSWERS

1. **a.** 3.
   b. 2.
   c. 1.
   d. 4.
2. Supine.
3. Any of the following: color, turgor, scars, lesions, hernias, superficial vessels, spider nevi, abnormal hair distribution, ascites, contusions, ecchymotic areas, burns/bruises.
4. Auscultation; percussion or palpation.
5. Normoactive.
6. False. Bowel sounds may be present even with an intra-abdominal injury.
7. Amount, odor, color, consistency, pH.
8. Drops.
9. Dehydration, electrolyte imbalance.
10. Nausea/vomiting.
11. Hemorrhage; perforation.
12. Resuscitation.
13. Arteriography does not visualize venous circulation.
14. Endoscopy.
15. Pancreatitis.
16. Amylase, lipase, CBC, glucose.
17. Assure patency; irrigations.
18. Pain; amylase or lipase.
19. Paralytic ileus.
20. Appendicitis.

21. Pain; McBurney's point.

22. Small; adhesions.

23. Hyperactive.

24. Will not reduce with gentle pressure.

25. Urinary retention; inguinal.

26. Motionless.

27. Determining whether or not surgery is needed.

28. a. 3.
   b. 4.
   c. 5.
   d. 6.
   e. 1.
   f. 2.

29. a. 2.
   b. 1.
   c. 4.
   d. 3.
   e. 5.

30. d. None of the above.

31. Patient cannot swallow.

32. 5 to 36.

33. 0.1 to 1.2 mg/dl.

34. False. An altered level of consciousness is an indication for peritoneal lavage.

35. Urinary catheter; gastric decompression tube.

36. Endoscopy.

37. Abdominal cramps.

38. Hemorrhage; intestinal rupture.

39. Retained barium/impaction; reaction to contrast medium.

40. Any of the following: destruction of bacteria, old RBCs, and platelets; production of lymphocytes and plasma cells; storage/release of blood.

41. Peptic ulcer disease.

42. Decreases mesenteric blood flow and in turn reduces portal hypertension.

43. Reduce pain.

44. ≥ 5.

45. Any of the following: paralytic ileus, infection, hemorrhage, coagulopathy, peritonitis, dehiscence, evisceration, retroperitoneal hematoma, respiratory involvement, pancreatitis.

SELECTED READINGS

Books

Bates B: *A Guide to Physical Examination*. Philadelphia: Lippincott, 1979

Bockus HL: *Gastroenterology*, vol. 1. Philadelphia: Saunders, 1974

Brunner LS, Suddarth DS: *Lippincott Manual of Nursing Practice*. Philadelphia: Lippincott, 1982

Cowley RA, Dunham CM: *Shock Trauma – Critical Care Manual*. Baltimore: University Park Press, 1982

Daly BJ: *Intensive Care Nursing*. New York: Medical Examination, 1980

Dykes PW, Keighley MRB, eds: *Gastrointestinal Hemorrhage*. Littleton, Ma: Wright-PSG, 1981

Eckert C: *Emergency Room Care*. Boston: Little, Brown, 1976

Friedman HH: *Problem-Oriented Medical Diagnosis*. Boston: Little, Brown, 1979

Gitnick G: *Handbook of Gastrointestinal Emergencies*. New York: Medical Examination, 1982

Givens BA, Simmons SJ: *Gastroenterology in Clinical Nursing*. St. Louis: Mosby, 1975

Govoni LE, Hayes JE: *Drugs & Nursing Implications*. New York: Appleton-Century-Crofts, 1978

Jeejeebhoy KN: *Gastrointestinal Diseases – Focus on Clinical Diagnosis*. New York: Medical Examination, 1980

Kenner CV, Dossey BM, Guzzetta CE: *Critical Care Nursing: Body-Mind-Spirit*. Boston: Little, Brown, 1981

Kinney MR: *AACN's Clinical Reference for Critical Care Nursing*. New York: McGraw-Hill, 1981

Koretz RL: *Practical Gastroenterology*. New York: Wiley, 1982

Miller MA, Leavell LC: *Anatomy & Physiology*. New York: Macmillan, 1972

Read AE, Harvey RF, Naish JM: *Basic Gastroenterology*, 3rd ed. Littleton, Ma: Wright-PSG, 1981

Reller LB, Sahn SA, Schrier RW: *Clinical Internal Medicine*. Boston: Little, Brown, 1979

Rice HV: *Gastrointestinal Nursing*. New York: Medical Examination, 1978

Seward C, Mattingly D: *Bedside Diagnosis*. New York: Churchill Livingstone, 1979

Sharp EH: *Handbook of General Surgical Emergencies*. New York: Medical Examination, 1977

Skydell B, Crowder AS: *Diagnostic Procedures*. Boston: Little, Brown, 1975

Sleisenger MH, Fordtran JS: *Gastrointestinal Disease*. Philadelphia: Saunders, 1973

Spivak JL, Barnes HV: *Manual of Clinical Problems in Internal Medicine.* Boston: Little, Brown, 1978

Tilkian SM, Conover MH: *Clinical Implications of Laboratory Tests.* St. Louis: Mosby, 1975

Periodicals

Jeejeebhoy KN: Low down GI bleeding. *Emerg Med* 14(7): 207, 213, 1982

Kadir S, Ernst CB: Current concepts in angiographic management of gastrointestinal bleeding. *Curr Prob Surg* 20:287, 1983

Mengel A: Getting the most from patient interviews. *Nursing 82* 12(11):47, 1982

Reber HA: Aid for the ailing pancreas. *Emerg Med* 14 (4): 94, 1982

INDEX

A

Abdominal distention
  hernias, 93
  mechanical bowel obstruction, 91
  paralytic ileus, 83
  vasopressin, 128
Abdominal drains. *See* Drains
Abdominal examination. *See*
  Assessment
Abdominal girth, paralytic ileus, 84
Abdominal trauma, 64-70. *See also*
  Penetrating wounds; Trauma
  abscess and, 70-71
  assessment, 64-69
  complications in, 70-74
  dehiscence and, 71
  diagnostic problems in, 64
  evisceration and, 71
  hemorrhage and, 70
  nursing considerations in, 68-70
  pancreatitis and, 73
  paralytic ileus and, 72-73
  peritonitis, 97
  primary peritonitis, 72
  respiratory involvement in, 73-74
  retroperitoneal hematoma and, 72
  wound infection and, 71
Abdominal wall puncture, 97
Abscess(es)
  abdominal wall trauma, 70-71
  appendicitis, 90
  cholecystitis, 94, 96
  mechanical bowel obstruction, 90
  needle-catheter jejunostomy, 116
  pancreatitis and, 79
  peritonitis, 98
Acid-base balance
  diarrhea, 48
  gastrointestinal bleeding, 58
  nausea/vomiting, 45
  paralytic ileus, 82-84
  Salem sump, 104
Acinar cells, 6
Addisonian crisis, 43
Adynamic ileus. *See* Paralytic ileus

Age
  appendicitis, 88
  cholecystitis, 94
  endoscopy, 136
  hernias, 93
  peptic ulcer disease, 53
Alanine aminotransferase (ALT). *See*
  Serum glutamic-pyruvic transaminase (SGPT)
Albumin, liver and, 10
Alcohol abuse
  abdominal trauma, 64
  consent forms, 69
  esophageal trauma, 62
  pancreatitis, 73, 78, 82
  peptic ulcer disease, 53
Alimentation. *See* Feeding
Alkaline phosphatase (ALP), 147
  abdominal trauma, 69
  cholecystitis, 95
  pancreatitis, 80
ALP. *See* Alkaline phosphatase
ALT. *See* Serum glutamic-pyruvic
  transaminase
Aluminum hydroxide gels
  (Amphojel), 129
Ambulation
  appendicitis, 90
  hernias, 94
  paralytic ileus, 83
Amphojel (aluminum hydroxide
  gels), 129
Ampulla of Vater, 6, 7, 10
Amylase levels
  abdominal trauma, 69
  cholecystitis, 95
  nausea/vomiting, 43
  pancreatic injury, 67
  pancreatitis, 80, 82
Analgesics
  appendicitis, 89
  cholecystitis, 96
  hernias, 94
  pancreatitis, 80, 82
Anaphylaxis. *See* Shock

Anemia, 80
Anesthesia
  nausea/vomiting, 43
  paralytic ileus, 82
Angiography
  esophageal trauma, 63
  gastrointestinal bleeding, 57
Antacids, 37, 39, 129-130
  cimetidine interactions, 129
  paralytic ileus, 84
Antibiotic therapy. *See also*
    Pharmacology
  appendicitis, 89-90
  cholecystitis, 95
  diarrhea, 48
  mechanical bowel obstruction, 92
  peritonitis, 98
Antiemetics, 37, 39, 44, 45. *See also*
    Pharmacology
Antispasmodics, 37, 39
Appendicitis, 88-90
  assessment, 88-89
  diagnosis/treatment, 89
  etiology, 88
  nausea/vomiting, 43, 44
  peritonitis, 97
  postoperative nursing considera-
    tions, 89-90
  preoperative nursing considera-
    tions, 89
Appendix, 2, 5
  assessment, 27
  barium enema, 141
Arrhythmias. *See also* Heart
  vasopressin, 128
Arterial blood gases. *See* Blood
    gases
Ascites
  appendicitis, 89
  pancreatitis, 79, 80
  peritonitis, 97
Aspartate aminotransferase (AST).
    See Serum glutamic-oxaloacetic
    transaminase (SGOT)
Aspiration pneumonia. *See*
    Pneumonia
Aspirin, 62

Assessment, 25-40
  abdominal trauma, 64-69
  appendicitis, 88-89
  auscultation, 28-29
  cholecystitis, 94-95
  diarrhea, 46, 47
  esophageal trauma, 62-63
  gastrointestinal bleeding, 54, 55
  inspection, 26-27
  mechanical bowel obstruction,
    90-91
  nausea/vomiting, 42-45
  palpation, 30-35
  pancreatitis, 78-80
  paralytic ileus, 83
  percussion, 30
  recovery postoperative phase,
    35-39
AST. *See* Serum glutamic-
    oxaloacetic transaminase
    (SGOT)
Atelectasis, 73
Atrial fibrillation, 137
Atropine, 48
Auscultation. *See also* Bowel sounds
  abdominal trauma, 64
  assessment, 28-29
  pancreatitis, 73
  paralytic ileus, 72-73
  respiratory involvement, 74
  Salem sump, 103
Automobile accidents, 64, 66, 67
Autonomic nervous system, 12

B

Back, palpation of, 35, 36
Bacteria. *See also* Infection;
    Sepsis
  liver, 10
  spleen, 13
Barium
  mechanical bowel obstruction,
    90, 91
  upper gastrointestinal series, 140
Barium enema, 141-142
Baseline laboratory studies. *See*
    Laboratory studies

Beta cells, 6
Bicarbonate, 6
Bile
  gallbladder, 11
  liver, 10
  small intestine, 5
Bile canaliculi, 10
Biliary tract disease, 78
Bilirubin, 148. *See also* Blood test
  abdominal trauma, 69
  cholecystitis, 95
  pancreatitis, 80
Bladder. *See* Gallbladder; Urinary
    bladder
Blood
  bilirubin, 148
  prothrombin time, 148-149
  spleen, 13
Blood count. *See* Blood test
Blood flow, liver, 8-10
Blood gases, 80, 81
Blood infection, 97
Blood pressure. *See* Hypertension;
    Hypotension
Blood test. *See also* Red blood cells;
    White blood cells
  duodenal injury, 67
  liver injury, 66
  mechanical bowel obstruction,
    91, 92
  nausea/vomiting, 43
  pancreatitis, 82
  small bowel injury, 66
  spleen injury, 65
Blood transfusions
  abdominal trauma, 68
  gastrointestinal bleeding, 59
  hemorrhage and, 70
Blunt trauma. *See* Abdominal
    trauma; Trauma
Body temperature. *See also* Fever
  abdominal trauma, 68
  cholecystitis, 96
  peritonitis, 98
Body weight, 18, 21
Bone, 147
Bowel function, 17-18, 20-21

Bowel ischemia/infarct, 82
Bowel rupture
  colonoscopy, 138
  sigmoidoscopy, 139
Bowel sounds
  abdominal trauma, 72
  auscultation, 28
  colonic injury, 66
  diarrhea, 46
  mechanical bowel obstruction, 91
  paralytic ileus, 72-73, 83
  peritonitis, 97
Bradycardia, 128
Breathing. *See also* Respiratory
      failure; Respiratory involvement
  palpation and, 32
Bronchial constriction, 128
Brunner's gland, 4, 5
Burns, 53

C

Caffeine, 53
Calcium, 80, 82
Calcium carbonate
      (Titralac), 129
Cancer
  gastrointestinal bleeding, 52
  mechanical bowel obstruction, 90
  pancreatitis, 78
Cantor tube, 106-108
Carcinoma. *See* Cancer
Cardiac glands, 4
Cardiac sphincter, 42
Cathartics, 37, 39
Catheters. *See also* Foley catheter;
      Needle-catheter jejunostomy
  intravenous, 68
CBC. *See* Blood test
Cecum, 2, 5
  barium enema, 141
Celiac ganglion, 12
Central nervous system trauma, 53
Central venous pressure, 68
Cholangiography, 80
Cholecystitis, 94-96
  assessment, 94-95
  complications, 96

I

Iatrogenic injury, esophageal
   trauma, 62
Iced lavage, 59
Ileocecal valve, 4,5
Ileum, 4
Ileus. *See* Paralytic ileus
Iliac crest, 5
Impaction. *See* Fecal impaction
Incarcerated (strangulated) hernia,
   35, 93. *See also* Hernias
Incisional hernias, 93. *See also*
   Hernias
Incisions, 37, 38
Indigestion, 94
Infection. *See also* Sepsis
   abdominal trauma, 70-71
   appendicitis, 88
   cholecystitis, 95
   Daval sump, 124
   diarrhea, 46
   Hemovac drainage system, 119
   pancreatitis, 78
   Penrose drain, 118
   peritonitis, 97
   Saratoga sump, 123
   Shirley sump, 121
Inferior mesenteric ganglion, 12
Inflammatory bowel disease
   diarrhea, 46
   mechanical bowel obstruction, 90
Infusion pump
   mercury-weighted feeding tubes,
      114
   needle-catheter jejunostomy, 115,
      116
Inguinal hernias, 93, 94. *See also*
   Hernias
Inspection
   abdominal trauma, 64
   assessment, 26-27
Insulin, 6, 7, 82
Intestinal glands, 4, 5
Intestinal obstruction. *See* Paralytic
   ileus
Intestinal secretion disorders, 46
Intestinal tubes. *See also* Drains;

Tubes
   mechanical bowel obstruction, 92
   paralytic ileus, 72, 83
Intestines. *See also* Colon; Small
   intestine
   alkaline phosphatase, 147
   percussion, 30
Intravenous catheters, 68
Intravenous cholangiography, 95
Intravenous (IV) therapy
   mechanical bowel obstruction, 92
   peritonitis, 98
Iron, 10
Ischemia, 90
Islets of Langerhans, 6, 7

J

Jaundice
   alkaline phosphatase, 147
   bilirubin, 148
   pancreatitis, 79
Jejunum, 4, 5

K

Kaolin, 48
Kaopectate, 48
Kehr's sign, 65
Kidney
   assessment, 27
   lactic dehydrogenase, 147
   palpation, 34
   serum glutamic-oxaloacetic trans-
      aminase, 146
Kupffer cells, 10

L

Laboratory studies, 145-149. *See also*
   Blood test
   abdominal trauma, 69, 72
   alkaline phosphatase, 147
   appendicitis, 89
   bilirubin, 148
   cholecystitis, 95, 96
   diarrhea, 47
   esophageal trauma, 63
   gastrointestinal bleeding, 54
   lactic dehydrogenase, 147

Prothrombin time, 148-149
Proximal colon, 12
Pseudocyst, 79
Psychosocial history, 19, 22. *See also* Patient history
PT/PTT. *See* Blood test
Pulse, 68. *See also* Vital signs
Pyloric sphincter, 27
Pyloric valve, 3, 4
Pylorus, 3, 42

R

Radiation therapy, 43, 44
Radiology
   barium enema, 141-142
   cholecystitis, 95
   diarrhea, 48
   esophageal trauma, 62, 63
   mechanical bowel obstruction, 91
   mercury-weighted feeding tube, 114
   Miller-Abbott tube, 110
   nausea/vomiting, 43
   pancreatitis, 79-81
   paralytic ileus, 83
   upper gastrointestinal series, 140
   vasopressin, 128
Reabsorption, 6
Rectal tubes
   diarrhea, 49
   paralytic ileus, 83
Rectum, 2, 5
   diarrhea, 47
   innervation, 12
Red blood cells. *See also* Blood; Blood test
   lactic dehydrogenase, 147
   liver, 10
   serum glutamic-oxaloacetic transaminase, 146
Respiratory distress, Salem sump, 103
Respiratory failure
   paralytic ileus, 82
   peptic ulcer disease, 53
Respiratory involvement
   abdominal trauma, 68, 72-74

endoscopy, 137
mechanical bowel obstruction, 92
pancreatitis, 79, 81
peritonitis, 98
Resuscitation, 58
Retching, 42, 62, 63. *See also* Nausea/vomiting
Reticuloendothelial system, 11
Retroperitoneal hematoma
   abdominal trauma, 72
   paralytic ileus, 82
Retroperitoneal pancreatic hemorrhage, 80
Rib fracture, 65, 66
Riopan (magaldrate), 129
Roentgenograms. *See* Radiology
Round ligament, 10

S

Salem sump, 102-104
   gastrointestinal bleeding, 54
Salivation, 42
Saratoga sump, 121-123
Seat belts, automobiles, 26, 28, 66
Semi-Fowler's position, 73, 81
Sengstaken-Blakemore tube
   gastrointestinal bleeding, 59
Sepsis. *See also* Infection
   mechanical bowel obstruction, 91, 92
   paralytic ileus, 82
   peptic ulcer disease, 53
Serum amylase. *See* Amylase levels
Serum glutamic-oxaloacetic transaminase (SGOT), 146
   abdominal trauma, 69
   cholecystitis, 95
   pancreatitis, 80
Serum glutamic-pyruvic transaminase (SGPT), 146-147
   abdominal trauma, 69
   cholecystitis, 95
Serum lipase. *See* Lipase levels
Sex differences
   cholecystitis, 94
   esophageal trauma, 62
   hernias, 92

OTHER VOLUMES IN THE

RN

NURSING ASSESSMENT SERIES

For information, write to:

Medical Economics Books
680 Kinderkamack Road
Oradell, New Jersey 07649